Eurythmy and Rudolf Steiner

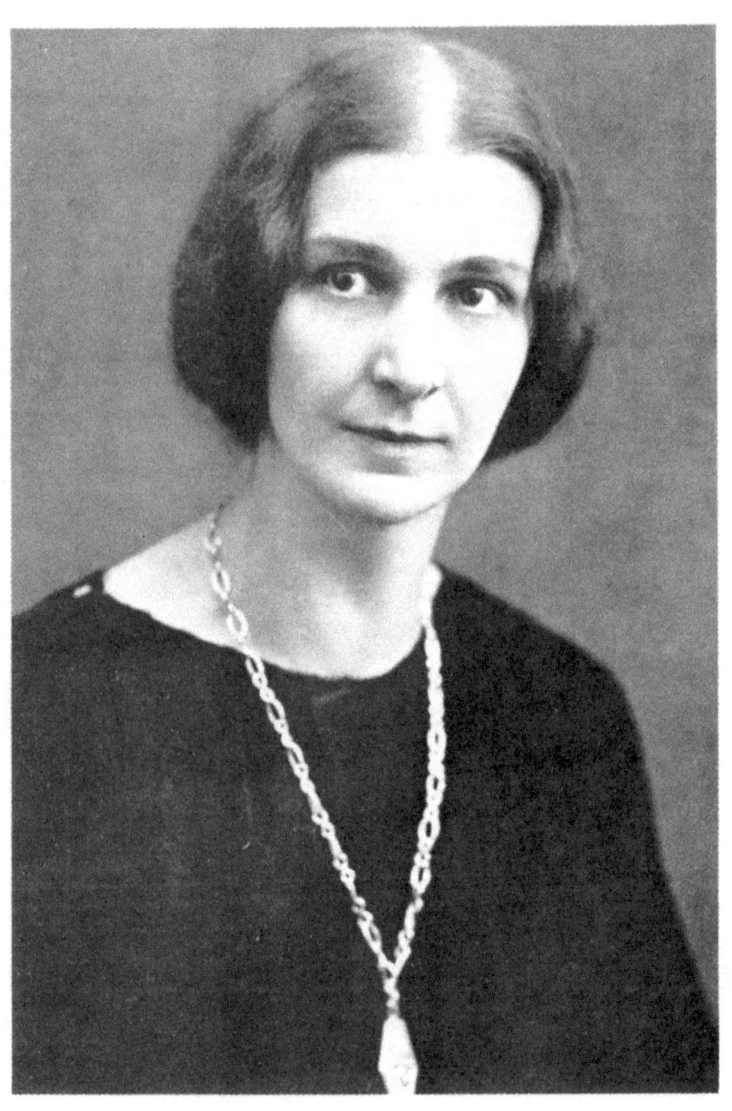

Tatiana Kisseleff, 1924.

Eurythmy and Rudolf Steiner

Origins and Development 1912–39

Tatiana Kisseleff

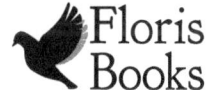
Floris Books

Translated by Dorothea Mier

Cover illustration © Daniel Hindes (www.eurythmyfigures.com)

First published in German as *Eurythmie, Erinnerungen aus den Jahren 1912–17*
by Waldhaus-Verlag Malsch in 1949, and *Aus der Eurythmie-Arbeit* (a supplement)
by Pforte Verlag in 1965
Published together as *Eurythmie-Arbeit mit Rudolf Steiner, Die Jahre 1912–1925*
by Pforte Verlag in 1982
First published in English by Floris Books, Edinburgh in 2021
© 1982 Futurum Verlag (Pforte Verlag)
English version © 2021 Floris Books

All rights reserved. No part of this book may
be reproduced without prior permission of
Floris Books, Edinburgh
www.florisbooks.co.uk

 Also available as an eBook

British Library CIP data available
ISBN 978-178250-738-3
Printed in Great Britain by CPI Group (UK) Ltd, Croydon

 Floris Books supports sustainable forest management
by printing this book on materials made from wood that
comes from responsible sources and reclaimed material

Contents

Introduction		7
Author's Preface		12
1912–13:	Foundation and Beginnings	15
1913–15:	Building Up	31
1915–18:	Expansion and Deepening	77
1918–19:	Stepping Out in Public	96
1919:	On Tour	122
1919–24:	In the House of the Word	128
1924–27:	Rudolf Steiner's Death – A Turning Point in My Life	141
1927–39:	Paris – Studio rue Huyghens and the École Rudolf Steiner	151
The Future of Eurythmy		183
Endnotes		206
Selected Bibliography		212
Index		213

Introduction

Tatiana Kisseleff was born in Warsaw on March 15, 1881, the daughter of Russian parents. She grew up with her older sister and younger brother in a family influenced by the arts and sciences. Her maternal grandfather was president of the Imperial Academy of Sciences, and his interest in Goethe's worldview lent his academic interests a universal quality: he was as at home in the sciences as he was in the arts and the religious sphere. Tatiana's mother was an energetic and imaginative woman who taught her children painting, literature and music.

While she was still very young, Tatiana's father, a colonel in the czar's army, died. Tatiana remembered how, shortly before he died, this tender, kind-hearted man placed her on a table and danced with her to a barrel organ. Tatiana was a weak and sickly child and her mother said that she should dance if she wanted to be healthy. Another thread of destiny was woven into her life. After the death of her father, Tatiana's family moved to St Petersburg to be close to her mother's grandparents.

Despite the artistic influences of her childhood, as Tatiana grew up her interests were drawn increasingly to the social realm as a central motif of her destiny. In 1881, the year she was born, Czar Alexander II had been murdered, and, as a result of the autocratic, reactionary rule of his son Alexander III, Russia sank into social and political unrest. Out of her desire to work towards solving social questions Tatiana studied law at the University of Lausanne. During this time she also worked in experimental psychology, using artistic occupational therapy to treat and rehabilitate criminals at the Asylum Villejuif in Paris. This was pioneering work at the time and Tatiana was successful, but she eventually discontinued the work, unable to substantiate her results scientifically according to conventional opinion.

After receiving her diploma in 1908, Tatiana returned to her family in Russia and married the painter Nikolai Kisseleff. The years that followed in Moscow were tumultuous ones. It was the time of the symbolists, Tolstoy's death in November 1910 shook the idealists, and Socialist-Marxist tendencies were becoming increasingly pronounced. Tatiana immersed herself in the struggle for social and artistic renewal. While studying Solovyov, she continually felt the urge to translate what she was feeling into movement, but she did not know what to do with her arms. In the house where she lived there was an Isadora Duncan dance school, but an invisible force seemed to hold Tatiana back whenever she approached the entrance. There was something in the way the subjective expressiveness of the dance sought to seduce her feelings that made her hesitate.

The struggle between inner fulfilment and outer constraints soon took a toll on Tatiana's physical and mental health. She spent Christmas 1910 in the Taitzy Sanatorium, and was diagnosed the following year with tuberculosis and sent to the Swiss mountains. Tatiana's former doctor in Lausanne questioned the diagnosis, however, and on his advice she went to the sea instead of the mountains. Tatiana began to sense the guiding influence of the spirit and knew the true cause of her illness was a pressing life decision.

During her stay, Tatiana was given a theosophical book on reincarnation and karma by a group of ladies who invited her to Paris. There, Tatiana witnessed the founding of the Parisian Lodge of the 'Star of the East', the organisation set up by the Theosophical Society to promote the young Jiddu Krishnamurti as the new World Teacher and the reincarnation of Christ and the future Maitreya Buddha. But she was unimpressed with the enthusiasm it provoked.

It wasn't until she later received a copy of *Knowledge of the Higher Worlds* by Rudolf Steiner that Tatiana knew she had

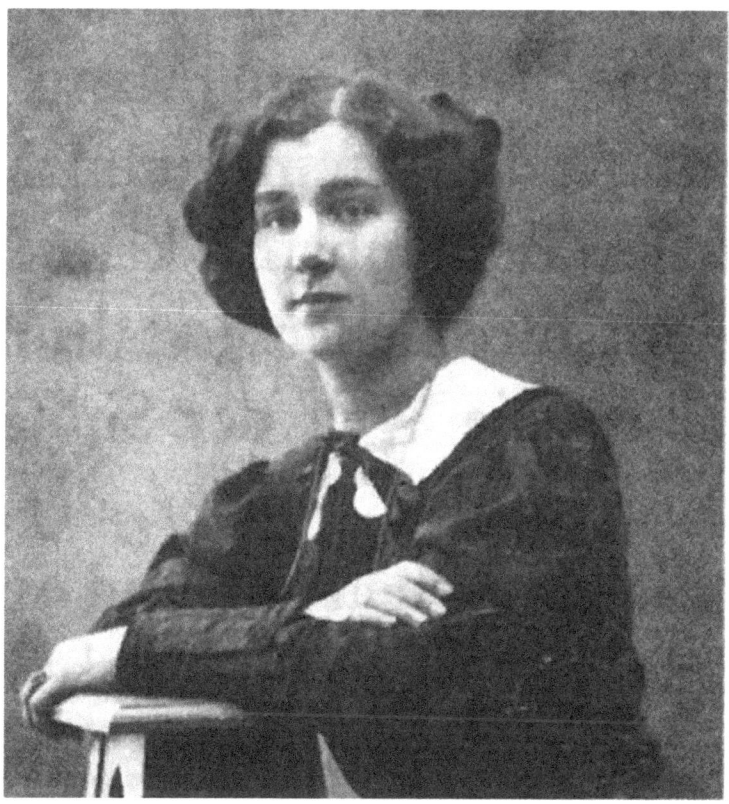

Tatiana Kisseleff as a student in 1904.

finally found what her soul was searching for. She travelled with her husband to Hanover where she became acquainted with Steiner and Marie von Sivers (later Marie Steiner).

It was Christmas, 1911; she was 30 years old.

Steiner accepted Tatiana as a personal student and directed her toward the art of eurythmy and away from the field of social services with which she was familiar. When she expressed doubt over this, mistrusting her deepest aspirations as arising out of personal desire, Steiner reassured her: 'You are an artist. You must trust yourself.' Tatiana was received into the Theosophical Society in Munich and subsequently moved to Düsseldorf to begin her artistic training. It was here that Lory (Maier) Smits was teaching the first students at the former monastery of Haus Meer.

Although exhilarating it was also a difficult time, one Tatiana characterised with lines from Rudolf Steiner:

> Life becomes lighter around me;
> Life becomes more difficult for me;
> Life becomes richer within me.

It is nevertheless impressive how short a time it took Tatiana Kisseleff, and many others, to grow into the practical life of anthroposophy under the guidance of Rudolf and Marie Steiner. A wealth of new revelations were taken up, and a certainty and faithfulness of spirit were cultivated in the face of the devastating conflict about to erupt in Central Europe.

Tatiana moved to Dornach just before war broke out in 1914 to teach the first eurythmy students, as well as the children of those working on the construction of the Goetheanum. Artistic activity was increasing and anthroposophical life in general was flourishing. Tatiana's tireless practising of the new art form, together with her deepening study of spiritual science, led to her most impressive creations. She mastered both serious and humorous subjects with equal perfection: from the performances of *Faust*, which took place during 1915–18, to humoresques written by Christian Morgenstern.

In 1919, Steiner brought eurythmy to the wider public with the first public performance in Zürich. In the years that followed there were many more public performances and lecture courses by Steiner, including the course on speech and tone eurythmy and on speech and drama. Tatiana witnessed this superhuman feat of work and commitment, before experiencing the pain of Steiner's death and the bitter struggles that ensued within the Anthroposophical Society.

During this time Tatiana had separated from her husband, although she remained connected to him. In 1927 she moved to Paris, where she taught eurythmy in a way that both engaged with French cultural life and also met the needs of Russian immigrants; she also worked on a eurythmy for the Russian language.

This was in fulfilment of Steiner's request that she bring eurythmy to Russia, although at the time that he made it he prevented her from returning to Russia due to the Russian revolution.

The Second World War paralysed all outer activity. Kisseleff spent this time in Dornach working on the chapters of this book that covered the years 1912–27, although it would not be published until 1949 thanks to the help of Tilla and Hubert Bollig. Throughout this time she was supported by Marie Steiner.

Through Tatiana Kisseleff, eurythmy, this art of the future, has today become a reality in the highest possible form. She is to be thanked for this valuable treasure, which we can do by taking seriously her reminder that the practice of eurythmy is inseparable from a path of self-development. She showed by example that one can use the etheric body just as one can use the physical; this was the fruit of her tireless work transforming everyday earthly consciousness into cosmic consciousness on the path indicated by Rudolf Steiner.

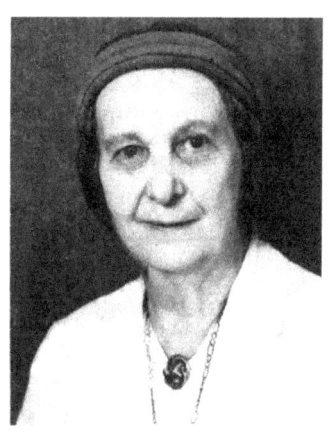
Tatiana Kisseleff in 1964.

Tatiana Kisseleff crossed the threshold in her ninetieth year on July 19, 1970. She had worked actively for three generations, and her teaching continues to live on in her many students.

Conrad Schachemann

Author's Preface

It has often happened that members of the Anthroposophical Society, especially many eurythmists who belong to the younger generation, ask me how eurythmy came into being, how it developed, and what it was like 'in earlier times'.

In spite of my wish to comply, so much has prevented me from describing in a comprehensive way, as I might in a conversation, all that I experienced in connection with the birth and development of eurythmy. But now it so happens that destiny has given me a period of time in which to carry out this work. After the many hardships and worries of previous years, I am now allowed to live for a while under the roof of the Carpenter's Shop in the immediate vicinity of the first Dornach stage and the hall in which Rudolf Steiner worked from 1913 until 1925. This was the scene of events that are never to be repeated and that are significant not only for that time but for the unforeseeable future.

Vivid images of the past rise up before my soul with incredible liveliness, and it is as though what once was still fills this space, as though the events that took place here are imprinted here for eternity. So I will attempt to fulfil the wish of the new generation, although I am fully aware of how weak and pallid the descriptions called up in their souls will be in comparison to the power and vibrant colour of the reality I actually lived through.

Added to the 1949 edition

Ten years have passed since I wrote down these memories. They had to wait a long time until they could find their way into the world in book form.

From a heart filled with deep, reverent gratitude towards Rudolf and Marie Steiner, I have decided that this memoir, intended at first for only a small circle, should be made available to all who are interested in this aspect of the anthroposophical spiritual stream.

The creators and teachers of the art of eurythmy are no longer physically among us. Rudolf Steiner only lived until March 30, 1925, two years after the burning of the Goetheanum, the greatest work of art of that time, which was destroyed on New Year's Eve 1922 by forces hostile to the spiritual progress of mankind.

Marie Steiner, who since the beginning of the twentieth century shared unspeakable hardships as the active, creative companion of this pioneering spirit, this guide to the heights of being, continued her activity in the service of spiritual work for more than twenty-three years after his death. She worked tirelessly to realise the transcendent goals of Rudolf Steiner until the end of her earthly life just a couple of months ago at the age of eighty-one. The most mature wisdom radiated through her in the many forewords she wrote for the lecture cycles, as well as through her own many essays and articles about art and other cultural concerns. Marie Steiner was gifted with a deep connection to speech formation, recitation, declamation and drama from her earliest youth. She dedicated herself to this art with great enthusiasm and its cultivation became one of her most important activities within the Anthroposophical Society. Later, especially after 1924, she devoted herself to the teaching and furthering of her countless students in the field of speech formation and the dramatic art and offered them the ripe fruits of her life's work.

May the art of eurythmy and the thoughts of the present

and future generations always be linked with the names of these two great helpers of humanity in their spiritual ascent. May seeds sown in all parts of the world find a fertile soil; that is, open human souls enthusiastic for true beauty and purity, who selflessly take up and nurture this seed and see that it is introduced into many centres of education. The development of artistic activity can protect against dangers of the present and in time to come. As with everything that has been brought to life and left to us by Rudolf Steiner and Marie Steiner in such a selfless way, so too eurythmy can become a nourishment for every human being who cultivates it with devotion. It can become the spiritual bread of life.

Tatiana Kisseleff
September 1939 and February 1949
Dornach

1912–13:
Foundation and Beginnings

In the years before the Great War a new creative impulse, founded in the life of the spirit, arose in Dornach just south of Basel in Switzerland. It was here, in the foothills of the Jura mountains, that people from many different nations were brought together by destiny to work on the building that was intended to be the outer expression of this new cultural-spiritual stream: the Goetheanum, at the time still known as the Johannesbau. Later, as war raged and humanity stood in shock before the ruins of a collapsing culture, the work carried out here served as a bulwark against the destruction and chaos unfolding all around them. And all of this was made possible because there lived and worked among us someone who, through mighty and inspiring cultural impulses, was

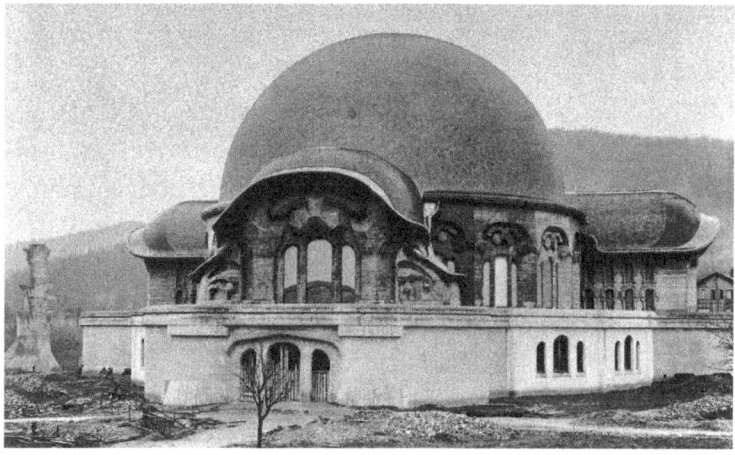

The first Goetheanum in Dornach, Switzerland, which burned down on New Year's Eve, 1922.

bringing the future to birth: Rudolf Steiner. The manifold and unending richness of all he gave us, day by day, until the last hours of his life, is incalculable.

It is my intention to present one aspect of this creative activity with which I am strongly connected through destiny, and to which I have dedicated my whole life since I first encountered it: the art of eurythmy.

In a certain sense eurythmy is both very old and very young, at once the first and the last artform to emerge in the succession of the arts. In the ancient mystery centres, a sacred art of dance and speech was practised that represented the spiritual forces behind the movement of the stars. At that time it was known that human beings journeyed through the starry realms before birth and that they had been created by exalted spiritual beings from out of the forces of the whole cosmos. In the temple dances, the movements of the stars were portrayed, bringing to expression humanity's connection to the whole universe. Later, other arts sprang out of these temple dances: sacred drama, sculpture, architecture, and poetry. But with the gradual loss of the original clairvoyance, human beings forgot the primal source from which the whole of culture originated. The dances became profane, inspired by passion and desire and embodying the subjective, arbitrary soul-life of the human personality. In this way, humanity became further estranged from the spiritual source of life.

In modern times, in place of the sacred art of movement, outdated expressions of Greek culture have been revived, such as the Olympic games. But these are purely external imitations and do not correspond to the needs of modern humanity.[1] Intellectual systems of dance have also arisen that have nothing to do with true art (there isn't the room to go into the nature and meaning of ballet here), and, in Asia, a few early traditions of temple dance have been preserved into the present in a beautiful but more or less rigid form. In Europe, a new guiding impulse was lacking.

That was the situation confronting Rudolf Steiner when he

brought forth his new art of movement. He called it eurythmy. It represents a renewal of the ancient art of the temple dance but in a completely modern form, one that acknowledges the change that has taken place in the physical and soul-spiritual constitution of modern humanity, and the new realities that prevail in the spiritual world at the present time. Out of this awareness, eurythmy strives to unite human beings once again with their spiritual home.

Rudolf Steiner says the following about how he came to this creation:

> The development of the art of eurythmy is based on the supersensible understanding of the expressive possibilities of movement in the human body. There is only a scant tradition of this understanding – as far as I know – still available from earlier times when the soul-spiritual nature shone through the physical body to a far greater extent than today. This meagre tradition, which incidentally indicates quite a different intention than that which is in eurythmy, was quite naturally used. But it needed to become independent and transformed and above all completely infused with the artistic. The manner of grouping people and moving them together in forms which has developed in eurythmy over time is not known to me out of any tradition.[2]

The dance of the luciferic and ahrimanic thought-beings (The Guardian of the Threshold)

Rudolf Steiner took the first step in reviving the ancient sacred art of dance in August, 1912, when he introduced the simple but extremely expressive dance of the luciferic and ahrimanic thought-beings from his third Mystery Drama, *The Guardian of the Threshold*.[3] At the invitation of Marie Steiner (who was then still Marie von Sivers), I entered the hall where the rehearsals were taking place. Many members of the Anthroposophical Society who were interested in Rudolf Steiner's new production had also been invited to participate in this initial work. Rudolf Steiner divided us into two groups. The first group, in which I was placed, had to form themselves together in curved formations (lemniscates and semi-circles) and make a gesture which expressed the spoken sound 'I' (*ee*). The second group were to move in pointed forms and make the gesture which corresponds to the speech sound '*A*' (*ah*).

These are the basic forms I drew according to Rudolf Steiner's directions:[4]

Luciferic thought-beings   Ahrimanic thought-beings

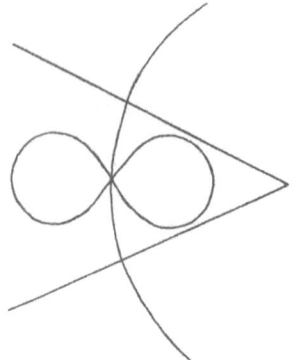 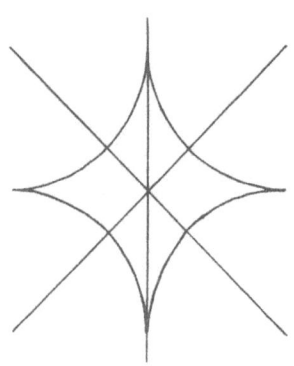

According to Rudolf Steiner's indications, the following phrases express the mood behind the formation of the different shapes, although the words were not spoken out loud.

For the luciferic beings: For the ahrimanic beings:

1. 'I will' – lemniscate   'I will' – square
2. 'I cannot' – curve   'I cannot' – straight line
3. 'I will' – lemniscate   'I will' – square
4. 'I must' – angle   'I must' – cross

The transitions from one position to the next were as follows:

Luciferic beings
For 1 and 2 (2 as position)   For 3 and 4 (4 as position)

Ahrimanic beings
For 1 to 4 (2 as position)

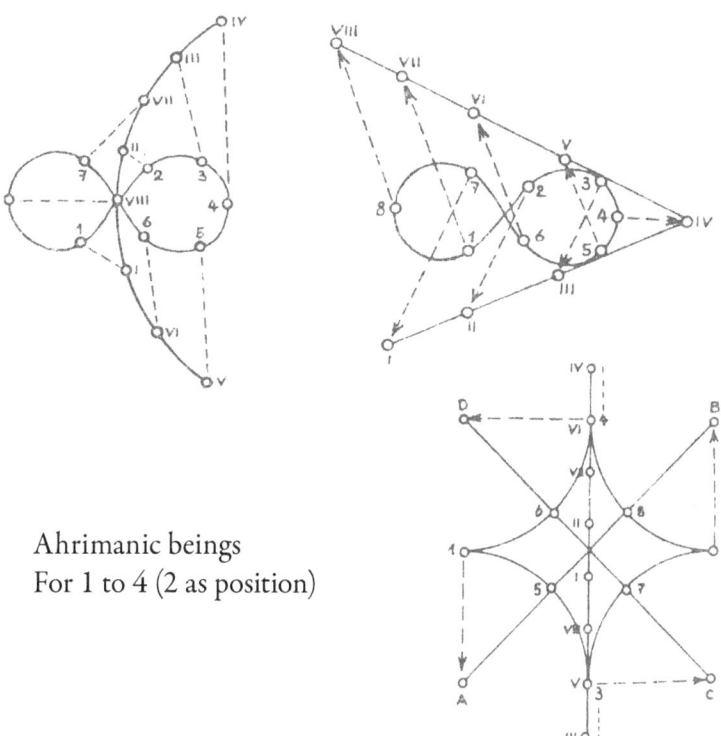

These short sentences were not performed as eurythmy. At that time no indication had been given for the sounds of speech other than the gestures expressing *I* for the luciferic beings and *A* for the ahrimanic beings. The luciferic beings wore red dresses with the addition of red-yellow wigs; the ahrimanic beings wore steel-blue dresses and wigs of the same colour. Dr Oskar Schmiedel gave signals from the prompter's box with an electric flashlight: red for the luciferic beings, blue for the ahrimanic beings. The transitions from one formation to the next, with eight people in each group, were a lot of hard work for us.

This work continued with the eurythmy course in Basel. There Rudolf Steiner gave the eurythmy gestures for all of the sounds of speech, the remaining vowels and the consonants, as well as the first eurythmy exercises and the so-called Dionysian forms: that is, more or less everything that is covered in the first year of a eurythmy course.

The Basel course

The first elements of a proper training in eurythmy were given the following month, in September 1912, in Basel, where Rudolf Steiner was giving a lecture cycle on the Gospel of St. Mark.

The outer reason for this first eurythmy course came from the following destiny situation. Frau Smits from Düsseldorf, whose daughter wanted to take up dance, asked for Rudolf Steiner's advice on the most suitable form. He provided the answer in the Basel introduction to eurythmy, which formed the basis for a schooling in a new art of movement.

In her foreword to *Eurythmy as Visible Speech* by Rudolf Steiner, Marie Steiner, who was asked to participate in these lessons, writes that:

> They contained the first elements of speech sound formation and a few exercises which belong largely to the pedagogical aspect of eurythmy: the basis for standing, walking, running, a few specific positions, many rod exercises, the gestures for expressing rhythm and rhythmic exercises. A few young ladies who were students of the first eurythmist developed the pedagogical aspect of eurythmy on this foundation. They then went over to working out the speech sounds of poems. That was the first phase of the eurythmy training.*

* This foreword is not included in the 2005 English edition.

I did not take part in the founding of eurythmy. I did not even know that the first lessons had taken place. But I would like to share an important experience I had at that time. Some readers may disapprove of this, but I am writing of my own personal memories, not a more general essay, and so I feel this may be permitted.

In the night that preceded the first instruction in eurythmy (which I discovered later by checking the entry in my diary), I had a kind of dream experience. I saw myself walking along a street in Basel when a car carrying Rudolf and Marie Steiner stopped in front of me. They invited me to join them on their further journey and so I got in. On arriving at their house they left me alone for a while in the anteroom. Suddenly the walls and ceiling vanished and I saw two human forms hovering in the air. They were dancing a most wonderful dance, hardly touching the ground as they simultaneously spread out into further rooms. I was deeply moved and excited by the sight of this unusual and sublime beauty. Throughout my whole youth, had I not always longed for a new, spiritual dance? Now I saw it fulfilled, even if it was only in a dream. With joyous animation, I told my companion at the hotel where we were staying about this strange experience. At the time, I had only been a member of the Anthroposophical Society for a few months, whereas my companion had been a member for longer. My dream appeared questionable to her. Rudolf and Marie Steiner dancing? That was impossible! She warned me that it might be a temptation and advised me to meditate thoroughly, especially before going to sleep. But I felt I had experienced a reality that I would come to understand only later.

The dance of the sylphs and gnomes (The Soul's Awakening)

A new and major event in the life of eurythmy was the performance, in August 1913, of the sylph and gnome dance in the then-new Mystery Drama, *The Soul's Awakening*.[5] Up until then, Rudolf Steiner had only given indications for individual movements. But now, during the rehearsal, he picked up two small sticks, bent down, and began to perform a gnome dance. He characterised the gnomes with such an astonishing mobility of his whole body and face that we looked on, speechless in amazement, as his familiar appearance vanished, replaced by a forcefully expressive gnome-like figure. What we are capable of expressing in eurythmy today is still very distant from what took place before our eyes on that occasion (see also p. 60, Rudolf Steiner as actor).

Rudolf Steiner's comments on eurythmy

Following this performance of *The Soul's Awakening*, Steiner gave a series of lectures in Munich called *Secrets of the Threshold*.[6] During this lecture cycle, on August 28, a small presentation of the elements of eurythmy and a few poems took place within the setting of a social gathering. Rudolf Steiner opened this with a few introductory words, as he often did in the following years before eurythmy performances.[7] He began with a conversation from one of the Mystery Dramas between Felicia Balde and Professor Capesius. Felicia is dissatisfied with the way Capesius listens to her fairy tales and says to him that if he were to listen properly, his etheric body would have to dance. When he asks how he could achieve this, she shares with him the source of her fairy tales. Capesius is astonished to hear that spiritual beings do not express themselves in any language existing on earth; instead they move, and one must learn to understand their movements. In answer to his question about how she does this, she says:

> One must understand art; one must allow the heart
> to rise up to the head for a while. Then one has a
> sense for all the movements which these elves, fairy

> tale princes, and fairies make, and what one then
> feels go like streams into the larynx. One can then
> retell this. Then if you listen properly, your etheric
> body should dance accordingly. As you are not able
> to do this, you are unable to understand everything
> and a lot of what I tell you gets lost.[8]

Rudolf Steiner continued:

> Now these communications of Frau Balde to
> Capesius have been taken, and it was tried – at least
> we have done it this way – systematically to bring
> out the movements of those elves, gnomes and
> also other dances of angels, into a kind of language
> movement.

He spoke further about Felicia's gifts:

> Frau Felicia was able to gaze out of the world of
> forms – which is the world of the physical plane
> – and to get glimpses into the world of the spirits
> of movement by allowing her heart to ray into her
> brain, even if unconsciously. And from there she
> received her fairy tales.

And he expressed the wish that people would approach this with the understanding that Capesius lacked.

> Now it would be quite nice, my dear friends, if ...
> with exchanges of thought also like those Frau Balde
> could bring out of the spiritual world, keeping a
> completely calm physical body, we could allow out
> etheric bodies to dance ... What we could establish
> in those meetings with Frau Felicia is now to form
> the basis of our art of eurythmy. The beginning
> should be made with an art which stands on a

borderland, and is consequently so meaningful. With the dance, you can express so to speak the most mundane things, that which lies nearest to the human instincts and passions. But it is also possible to embody the Dionysian element in the evolution of humankind.[9]

Rudolf Steiner indicated that a threefold intention lies behind eurythmy. The first is to give expression to the element of beauty. This is the direct expression, an intensification even, of what takes place in the higher worlds as something like movement: it is the aesthetic element. The second intention relates to the pedagogical or didactic element, and the third to the hygienic or therapeutic element. At the end of the address, he expressed the wish that 'our youth – those up to their sixtieth or seventieth year –would gain an understanding for this eurythmy'. And he added:

> When our youth will gradually become used to gaining an understanding for this expressive art, then there will be ever more people amongst us, to whom Frau Balde can say, 'You do not listen quite so badly anymore. You do already understand me better.'[10]

After a while the upper limit of these youthful years was pushed even further. As far as I know it happened on the following occasion. In Munich, whoever was able to among the members, signed up for an introductory course in eurythmy. The class was held in a small, narrow space and sometimes one had to wait a while before one's turn came because not everyone could move around the room at the same time, especially when one started to work on the Dionysian forms. We are told that an anthroposophist, on being invited to participate, answered sadly that he was over the permitted age: he was already seventy-two. I presume that Rudolf Steiner heard about this because sometime later, in a lecture he gave on October 7, 1914, he touched on the problem of age, saying:

> We might wish that humanity would be seized by an understanding of [eurythmy], so that it would be practised by children from the smallest, who have already experienced the most intimate joy from it, to the largest, and on up to people seventy, eighty, and ninety years old.

He added with a smile:

> It is always good when a person learns to transfer what is natural and inborn in the etheric body into physical movements.[11]

I will return to this lecture later.

A few more eurythmy presentations took place in the same year: in Leipzig by Erna van Deventer-Wolfram; in Cologne by the group working with Lory Smits, to which I also belonged; then two presentations in Berlin during the General Meeting of the Society in January 1914.

In the first presentation in Berlin, given by Erna van Deventer-Wolfram, texts in oriental languages, including Hebrew and others, were done in eurythmy accompanied by cymbals and the recitation of the original texts. The second presentation included texts in German and one in Russian and was presented by the Smits group. This preceded a lecture by Rudolf Steiner in which he spoke about the damage caused by the immobile, fixed thinking of modern humanity. He referred to the book *Contributions to the Criticism of Language* by Fritz Mauthner, characterising it as an outpouring of an endlessly tragic, rigid thinking. In contrast to Mauthner's pessimistic conclusions, Steiner developed his own positive conception out of an insight into the spiritual nature of the word and language. He said that out of the fount of the creative thoughts of the world, out of the source in which the Logos, the Word, is creatively active in the human etheric body, he had attempted to find the gestures that also express themselves outwardly in the resting human body, gestures that are imprinted not with what is dying in the human body (as Fritz Mauthner claimed) but with what is living.[12]

Steiner speaks in this lecture about the health-giving effect of the eurythmy gestures that extend to all the soul forces, so that from the etheric body the whole human being becomes penetrated with a healthy moral feeling and thinking: 'Thoughts will learn to move artistically. Then we will be standing before the redemption of humanity in this particular sphere.' Then Steiner drew our attention to the fact that eurythmy comes to meet the longing in human souls for a living, eternal source, while impotence in the realm of knowledge in our present age (the nineteenth and twentieth centuries) is plunging us into despair and illness.

Someone who was especially representative of this tragic longing of our time was Friedrich Nietzsche. He suffered so terribly from this symptom of longing that he became ill, the contemporary philosophy and worldview had infected his thoughts. His work, *Thus Spoke Zarathustra*, is a testament to the endless depth of his longing and his vague sense of the redemption of humanity. Nietzsche presents Zarathustra as an ideal of discernment, who tries to enliven human concepts, ideas and worldviews through a musical, dance-like quality: Zarathustra is a dancer. In almost exactly these words, Rudolf Steiner spoke about Nietzsche's ideals and longings at the end of his lecture.

The further development of the elements of eurythmy took place in 1912–13. This was done with the help of Frau Smits in her home at Haus Meer, near Düsseldorf, with her young daughter, Lory Maier-Smits, a few ladies and girls who gathered in her home, and the two younger sisters of Frau Smits as the first pupils.

My eurythmy notebook: corrections and indications from Rudolf Steiner

The notes for speech sounds and forms in my eurythmy notebook correspond to the lessons. During my eurythmy work with Marie Steiner at the end of summer 1914 in the Villa Hansi in Dornach (see the next chapter), Rudolf Steiner checked my movement of the vowels and consonants and asked to see my eurythmy notebook, which he kept for a few days before handing it back with corrections and other notes he had added. Since then, in teaching eurythmy, I have always kept to these indications. I showed them to Annemarie Dubach-Donath, Erna van Deventer-Wolfram, and also to Lory Maier-Smits when she visited me in 1960.

Rudolf Steiner told me that when doing the sound *U*, I did not always need to turn upwards. *U* could also be done downwards or forwards or sideways. What was important was that the arms were held parallel.

Regarding the diphthong *EI* he later remarked that the movement of the whole body should not be carried out in this way. Already in the first years of the development of eurythmy he no longer allowed this movement, but rather emphasised the movement of the arms and hands. Especially when doing eurythmy with poems in the Russian language, which has many *EI* and other related diphthongs (*AI, OI, UI*), we were not allowed to move our whole body. Instead we had to express these 'double sounds' exclusively through specific movements of the arms and hands.*

In the 1924 eurythmy course, Rudolf Steiner gave new indications. With words such as *'Eiapopeia'* or *'Lalobei'* (the equivalent of the English word 'lullaby'), and such words that

---

* The vowels A, E, I, O and U correspond approximately to English vowels in the following way: *A* as in *father*, *E* as in *gate*. *I* as in *me*, *O* as in *go*, and *U* as in *boot*, *Ä* as in *cat*, *AU* as in *cow*, *EU* as in *boy*, *EI* as in *my*, *Ö* as in *bird*. *ÄU* (like EU) as in boy, *Ü* as in the French *une*.

Pages from Tatiana Kisseleff's notebook on the vowel sounds in eurythmy with Rudolf Steiner's corrections (images slightly reduced from the original).

Tatiana Kisseleff's rendering of the text

My text		Rudolf Steiner's corrections
Resistance. Hands bent upwards.	A	Arms in an angle. Arms stay with hands. Shock; that which protects itself.
Crossing. Amazement (Reverence, Fear, Disgust).	E	'Amazement' crossed out; 'Reverence, Fear, Disgust' underlined.
Legs, hands placed one behind the other.	Ä	
Every stretch.	I	Indicating experiencing oneself in oneself.
Every touch of one's own body.	AU	'Touch' crossed out and replaced with 'press'.
Every bringing together. Rounding of the limbs. Lovingly embracing.	O	'Admiration' added.
Every turning upwards.	U	Crossed out. 'Both hands parallel, expressing wonder', added instead.
Jumping up or unity of the limbs.	ÄU	'Jumping up' crossed out. 'Jump with the touching of the floor afterwards' added instead.
Feel every movement of the whole body as 'How adorable!'	EI	'whole' underlined.
With hands placed on the heart or on the other hand, meaning the other, him.	EU	From the word 'or' onwards in on brackets and substituted with, pointing to 'With hand lying on the heart and an "as though" pointing arm'. For the speech sound EU he wrote, 'like "heu"'.
Round dance and jumping from a point into the centre. Also a sudden movement.	Ö	'towards the side' added.
The dancing past one another. The going past one another. Back of the hands. (Also feet next to each other.)	Ü	'Wonder with joy' added.

calm and lead a small child into sleep – *'Schlaf Kindlein ein'* ('Go to sleep, little child') – the experience of 'How adorable!' comes of its own accord and with it, quite naturally, the movement of the eurythmist's whole body.

In contrast, such words as *'Eis'* (ice), *'Eisen'* (iron), *'steif'* (stiff), and others that can hardly be felt as 'How adorable!', are best expressed through the movements of the arms and hands without the movement of the whole body.

1913–15: Building Up

Berlin beginnings

The laying of the foundation stone of the first Goetheanum took place on September 20, 1913. At the time, I was living in Berlin.

As Rudolf and Marie Steiner mostly lived in Dornach during the months following the laying of the foundation stone, I was able to give my first eurythmy lessons in their Berlin house at Motzstrasse 17. The pupils were a group of members of the Anthroposophical Society whom Mieta Pyle-Waller had brought together. These included Mieta herself, Olga von Sivers, Louise Carson, Frau Siedlecka, Miss Harris, and Mrs Ricardo. I was the teacher and also had to recite the texts. The big dining room was emptied of all furniture so that for a few months we could do eurythmy freely and enthusiastically. Some exercises were accompanied on the piano, with pianists Walter Kühne, a German who preferred Russian music, and Wladimir Papoff, a Russian who played German music, taking it in turns to play. Mathilde Scholl was always our audience.

After Christmas, Rudolf and Marie Steiner came to Berlin for a short while. Marie Steiner visited these lessons on two occasions and, before departing, expressed her satisfaction. After a few weeks, she suggested that I come to Dornach as a eurythmy teacher and give eurythmy lessons to the anthroposophists both there and in other places. On her recommendation, I took lessons on the art of speaking for a few weeks before departing for Dornach. These were with the well-known teacher, Frau Dietschi, who had been an actress at the end of the nineteenth century at the German Theatre in St. Petersburg. Marie Steiner thought very highly of the exercises she used in her introductory lessons, which helped her pupils achieve a melodious sound and accurate, precise pronunciation.

In Dornach: the Hotel Jura and the Villa Hansi

On March 30, 1914, I travelled to Dornach. On my arrival I found the Goetheanum, which at that time was provisionally called the Johannesbau, at the stage when it was customary to celebrate the so-called *Richtfest*, the topping-out or roofing ceremony. I saw trees decorated with many coloured ribbons on the wooden beams of the cupola, which was not yet covered with slate tiles. Next to it, in the Carpenter's Shop, work was in full swing. In the large space where the stage would later be built and where the lecture hall would come into being, there was nothing more than carpentry benches, blocks of wood and all sorts of tools. Shortly afterwards, Rudolf Steiner gave lectures in this space. We sat everywhere and anywhere, wherever one could find a space: on building material, on machines, on the floor.

Immediately upon my arrival in Dornach, I began to look for a room for eurythmy lessons. There was nothing to be found. I was growing desperate when one day, when I spoke about my difficulties to someone in the village, I was told to look at the rooms in the village pub, the Hotel Jura. (This pub does not exist anymore in its simple form as in those days; it has been enlarged and modernised.) The pub did indeed have a large room, with two little side rooms and an old, untuned piano. For thirty francs a month all of this was placed at my daily disposal from early morning until late at night. The only exceptions were Saturday afternoons and all of Sunday, when the village residents gathered for eating, beer drinking and entertainment.

Shortly afterwards the workings of destiny brought a musician into our circle: Adina Zinovsky from Reval,[*] who was on

---

[*] Reval is the ancient name of Tallinn, the capital of Estonia. The name was in official use in Estonia until 1918.

a journey from Italy to Russia, where she taught German language and literature. Adina came to Dornach intending to stay for only a few days, but when she heard that a pianist was needed for the eurythmy lessons she decided to remain and take on this position.

I once asked Rudolf Steiner what the best musical instrument to accompany eurythmy would be, and he replied that it would actually be a lyre, although a piano would do for the present moment. He promised to create a lyre with a new construction suitable for humanity's present stage of musical consciousness, but war broke out soon after and Steiner became too busy to realise these intentions.

At the entrance to the old canteen – in those days it was a simple wooden structure with a low roof, a few benches and tables in the small room and outside – we announced the beginning of eurythmy lessons. This was preceded by the reading of the lecture that Steiner gave in Bergen, Norway, about the different forces that enable human beings to perceive the spiritual world.[1] In connection with eurythmy, I mention only the following from the lecture. After many years of intensive work in eurythmy, at the very least after seven years, it is possible that those forces that are active in the human being in the first years of childhood, through which the child learns to stand upright, could be called to life. These are the purest, most innocent forces in human nature. After the first three years of life, these forces become ever more lamed, especially once school begins. If one succeeds in reviving these forces, they develop the capacity to see into those spiritual worlds that the soul inhabits between the last death and the birth into the present life: namely, the perception of that which happens in the spiritual world as the human being, together with the spiritual hierarchies, prepares their present earthly life. Bringing these experiences into consciousness has immense significance for a person's whole life on earth.

The following day, the first lesson took place, and the work that began then has continued ever since without stopping.

Certainly, it has met with many obstacles, but all have been overcome through those spiritual forces that belong to the very first beginnings of eurythmy. It happened once that we learned that a few men planned a protest against the 'dance at the place in which a building for the mysteries was being erected' and wanted to prevent our work. Because of their dark, everyday clothing, they were easy to spot as they sat together in one corner of the room. We eurythmists, women and men, were all dressed in white robes[2] and holding copper rods as we stood ceremoniously around the room. Without those present noticing anything, I turned to the pianist and requested that she fill every pause that might occur in my teaching with music. In that way, I hoped to prevent the men from protesting. But our fears proved unnecessary. After half an hour's practice, one of the men from the group of 'conspirators', obviously the initiator, approached me. With great emotion he confessed that he and his companions had intended to drive ourselves and our 'undesirable' dances out of Dornach, not thinking them compatible with the seriousness of things. But instead he expressed the overall enthusiasm of his whole group towards what they had just witnessed.

It became clear that these men had never before seen a eurythmy performance, nor heard Rudolf Steiner speak in his introductions about the importance of this art. And what they *had* heard from other members of the society had not been very convincing. This representative of the newly converted 'enthusiasts for anthroposophy in Dornach' subsequently became an especially keen and enthusiastic student of eurythmy! However, after only two or three weeks, he came to the lesson looking sad. The reason for his sadness, he explained, lay in the fact that his office work at the Goetheanum prevented him from taking part in eurythmy classes more than twice a week. He was concerned that because of this he would fall behind the others, who would be practising twice or three times as much, both artistically and anthroposophically.

When Rudolf Steiner heard of this, he explained that for the spiritual development of the human being, it did not matter what one did in the service of the spirit, be it typewriting, eurythmy or anything else. For him, a good office worker was just as valuable as a good eurythmist. Steiner went on to add that he personally liked typing far more than many other things he had to do.

Beyond this I do not wish to write much about the hindrances. There were many, especially in the first years of the work and then also later at the beginning of our eurythmy tours. But everywhere, ever and again, a corrective made its appearance sooner or later and the True and the Just triumphed.

Already in 1914, a few months after the beginning of the work, Marie Steiner took over the cultivation of eurythmy. We have her to thank for its rapid growth and many-sided development. In August and September of that year, eurythmy was practised every morning in the two rooms in the Villa Hansi, where Rudolf and Marie Steiner lived. Marie Steiner and I and sometimes Mieta Pyle-Waller took part. From time to time, Rudolf Steiner checked our work and each time he gave various new indications. The book *The Basic Principles of Eurythmy,* which Annemarie Dubach-Donath published, contains much of what was added to the course in Basel during this time.

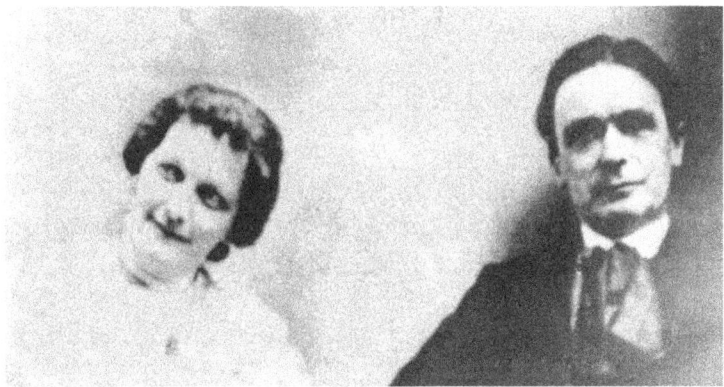

Rudolf and Marie Steiner on the balcony of the house in the Motzstrasse, Berlin, 1915.

Consonants in the sequence of human evolution (I)

On one occasion Rudolf Steiner took my book for a few days and wrote in additions, corrections, explanations and new elements. At that time, he wrote the order of the twelve consonants: *B, M, D, N, R, L, G, Ch, F, S, H, T.*

On the empty pages between my notations on the usual sequence of consonants, Rudolf Steiner wrote the sequence on the previous pages with these explanations:

BMDNRL – The human being seeking protection, becoming animated and calming down again

B – protected within something one becomes strong and can permeate. } *M*

B – the other
M – my attempt to go in
D – I myself

When you perform *B, M, D,* one after the other, then feel: Bei *ihm da* bin ich (With him, there am I).

For *CH* Rudolf Steiner made a drawing and wrote: 'as if fanning wind towards oneself.' I had not written this sound in the usual sequence.

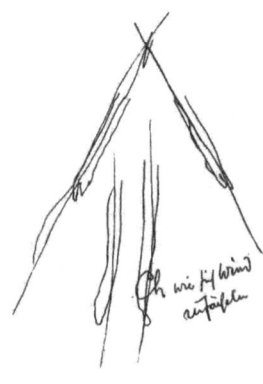

Pages from Tatiana Kisseleff's notebook with additions by Rudolf Steiner.

The corrections Rudolf Steiner made to the sequence I had written are:

B – as 'taking something in the hand' (rather than 'having') he added, 'I will be protected by something'.
D – he added: 'I must go through.'
M – for 'feel oneself in something', he crossed out 'in something' and added 'as though in the air'
N – he added: 'touch fleetingly'.
W – he remarked: 'vowel-like'.
L – he added: 'related to I'.
P – he added: 'in three'

Steiner explained that contained within this grouping of consonants was all that belongs to the development of humankind, and that if we worked properly in eurythmy with just these twelve sounds, then he would not need to give us his lectures. (He also said we could speak these sounds in this sequence without doing them in eurythmy.) He had already said something similar to this in connection with the Mystery Dramas, namely, that he would not need to hold any more lectures if people absorbed and understood the plays properly. This may be easier to understand when said of a play rather than the indications Steiner gave for the twelve consonants. His lecture cycle *Man in Light of Occultism, Theosophy and Philosophy* throws a strong light on this problem, especially the tenth lecture in which he mentions the twelve signs of the zodiac. These represent twelve mighty spiritual beings who speak of primeval times in cosmic and human evolution and through whom the original being of the Unspoken Word of Worlds speaks.[3] I point to further work in this direction in Consonants and the zodiac (p. 115).

Dance of the stars

Rudolf Steiner also spoke to us about the dance of the stars. He said that in earlier epochs there were many complicated dances that followed the laws of the fixed stars and planets and in which each planet performed its own path differently from the others. These dances represented sun and star eclipses, as well as many other things, and he wanted to revive and develop these dances when he had the time.

During one practice session where Marie Steiner, Mieta Pyle-Waller and I were present, Rudolf Steiner gave us an indication of these dances. As we performed spiralling movements, he recited verses based on specific sounds, creating them directly as he spoke. One verse represented the sun (Marie Steiner), the other the earth (Mieta Pyle-Waller), and the third the moon (Tatiana Kisseleff). Unfortunately, these verses were not written down, neither are they to be found in his posthumous works. This first dance of the stars that took place in Villa Hansi was only done once – on the day of its inception. Here is the form that I drew according to Rudolf Steiner's indications.

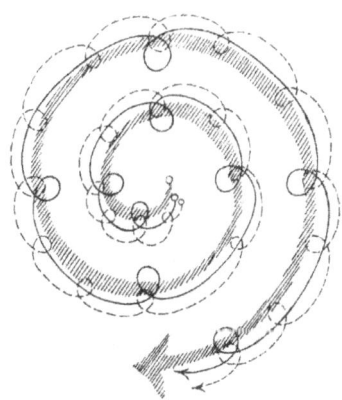

It is important therefore that we concern ourselves with the working together of these three 'stars', and we can perhaps do this best by considering the lecture cycle *Human and Cosmic Thought*, which Steiner gave in Berlin in 1914.[4] In the lecture of January 22, he characterises the twelve main worldviews, representing the spiritual element of the zodiac, and the seven soul moods, representing the spiritual element of the planets. He then points to the connection that exists between these two.[5] Furthermore, these worldviews can be 'modified yet again by possessing quite definite tones'.[6] Steiner then distinguished between three soul tones: theism, intuitionism, and naturalism. These have their replica in the outer world of the cosmos and behave in the human soul in the same manner as the sun, moon and earth, so that theism corresponds to the sun (the sun now seen as a fixed star), intuitionism corresponds to the moon, and naturalism to the earth. Further important explanations are contained in the final lecture of the cycle. I would also recommend the lecture Steiner gave in London on August 30, 1922, called 'The Other Side of Human Existence', where Christ is described as our guide through the manifold and bewildering events of the zodiac.[7]

Working in the Carpenter's Shop

In the autumn of 1914 we moved from the room in the Hotel Jura in the village into the Carpenter's Shop at the Goetheanum. To begin with, there was no heating and we warmed ourselves with eurythmical movements, and in the breaks we sat huddled in our coats. The floor was rough and sharp wood splinters kept tearing the soles of our thin eurythmy shoes and went into our feet. We waited with longing for the completion of the eurythmy room in the Goetheanum, but the work of eurythmy continued without interruption. Despite the fact that nearly all male workers had to leave Dornach, work on the building continued although at a slower pace. The Carpenter's Shop received one improvement after another: chairs appeared, followed by heating and, finally, the unforgettably joy of seeing the stage hung with blue curtains, which Steiner said corresponded mainly to the mood of Advent. Later on, different coloured curtains were added: white with bands of yellow for Christmas, black for the time before Easter, red for Easter itself, and mauve for Whitsun.

The first eurythmy lecture in Dornach

Rudolf Steiner spoke about eurythmy for the first time in Dornach on October 7, 1914. It was in connection with descriptions he gave of the remarkable and significant experiences undergone by the poet Christian Morgenstern, who had died that year at the end of March. Steiner said that in the spiritual world in which he presently resided, Christian Morgenstern had become a teacher and helper to many souls, including among them Herman Grimm. These souls were able to learn from him what they had not been able to find during their life on earth.[8]

In this lecture, Steiner spoke of how humanity in the last century longed for a new epoch of spiritual wisdom and experience, and how it stood at the threshold of what spiritual science now has to offer. The last representative of this epoch of expectation was Herman Grimm. In his soul lived a deep striving for spiritual truths and an understanding of the hierarchies; he yearned for the spiritualisation of the whole of life and longed for a new form of beauty to arise out of the fountainhead of the spirit. But Herman Grimm did not want a spiritual science that came to him in the form of abstract concepts. According to Steiner:

> Humanity has already striven to bring life into harmony with the spiritual worlds ... And that the offshoots of our spiritual movement should arise from the whole of our spiritual life should indeed be a fulfilment of expectation. So it is with eurythmy ... it was pulled out of our spiritual endeavours, so that people can learn especially in

this sphere how the spirit works in the most direct and intimate experience ... In brief, one can define eurythmy as the fulfilment of what the human etheric body demands from the human being according to its natural laws. Hence eurythmy really offers something that belongs to our spiritual life as well, and something that is thought out from its totality.[9]

Further notes by Rudolf Steiner

In my eurythmy notebook, under the drawing for the exercise *I and You*, Rudolf Steiner wrote, 'against conceit and egoism'.

For the exercise for *We*, he wrote, 'joy in being together'.

For the exercise for *He*, he wrote next to the word 'devotion', 'what one brings toward a Being'.

For the exercise for *You*, above the drawing of the harmonious eight he wrote, 'in order to cultivate harmony'.

For the spiral going from inside out he wrote, 'communication of strength'.

Rudolf Steiner also added a few drawings. For example, for the soul gesture *Ceremonious* in profile: 'Right arm with horizontal upper arm at shoulder level, lower arm and hand at right angle upwards, the left arm with upper arm against the body and lower arm and hand stretched horizontally forwards.'

For *Reverence*: 'Fold hands in *K*.' (*K* = *Kreuz* – cross.)

Next to the text *The Cloud Illuminator*: 'In order to develop the feeling and the mood of devotion and to acquire peace.'

For the exercise *You*, under the drawing of the lemniscate, he wrote, 'In order to cultivate healthy merriment.'

For *Piety*: 'Lifted folded hands'.

For *Devotion*: 'Flat hands laid on the breast with bent head'.

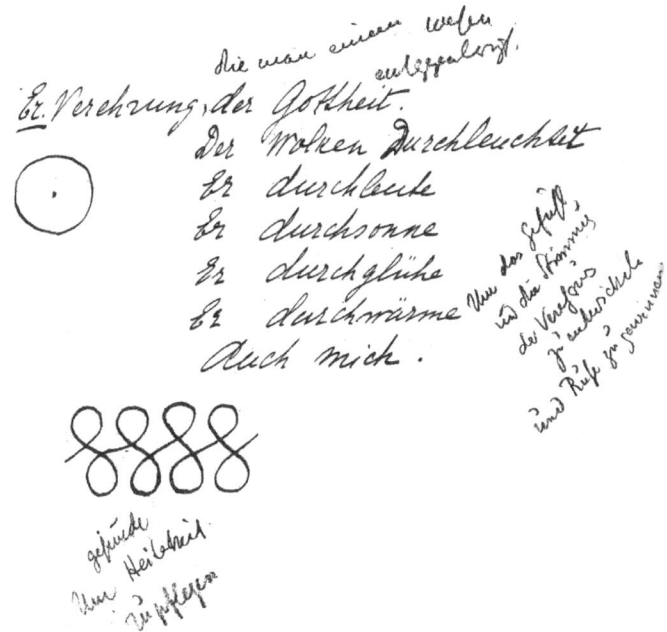

Reproduction of page from Tatiana Kisseleff's notebook, with additions by Rudolf Steiner.

Expressing vowels and consonants

I received the first suggestions for expressing vowels and consonants, aside from those I had already received for *Pater Noster* (see p. 62), from Rudolf Steiner in the late summer of 1914. These related to working with the soul forces in scene 7 of *The Portal of Initiation*. The indications for the sounds were:

— Philia = vowel-like (all vowels)
— Astrid = consonants
— Luna = both (vowels and consonants)

Already in 1915, Rudolf Steiner gave new directions so that no single sound was missing from the eurythmical presentation of this scene. This changed the distribution of the sounds somewhat, as the choruses were meant to fill out the gestures of the main soul forces expressed by the three characters. Philia's chorus did the consonants as a complement to her vowels; Astrid did all the vowels and a few consonants and the chorus added the rest; and Luna did all the consonants while the vowels were left to the chorus.

Rudolf Steiner's further comments related to poems. No poems, including those that express the interplay of inner soul conditions, should be done only with vowels: the whole word structure should be presented, all the speech sounds should be there. The consonants should not be allowed to fall away but must at least be indicated in the transition from one vowel to the next. In addition, poems that portray mostly outer events should not be done only with consonants, and the vowels likewise should be indicated in the transition from one consonant to the other. Only when practising is one allowed to do only the vowels or only the consonants in a poem, never in a performance. Steiner wanted eurythmy to serve as visible speech, to be a proper language, not just a babbling as with small children who cannot pronounce all the sounds in a word.

I will have more to say later about the justified and unjustified reduction of the number of sounds, as well as about performing them without rushing about.

The winter solstice verse: 'Behold the sun...'

Soon after Rudolf Steiner began giving lectures in the Carpenter's Shop of the Goetheanum in the autumn of 1914, members of the Anthroposophical Society suggested playing music as an introduction to his lectures. He rejected this, but instead requested that eurythmy be done before his lectures. Following this, for many months, I worked with two verses from the Calendar of the Soul and other verses by Steiner, performing them as eurythmy before lectures while Marie Steiner recited them. At Christmastime 1914–15, I performed the verse marking the winter solstice, 'Behold the Sun...', which Steiner had given in Berlin on December 17, 1906.[10] In due course other Dornach eurythmists also took part in these introductions.

Rudolf Steiner's indications for 'Behold the sun . . .' were as follows. A line indicates a step.

For-ward	*Die Sonne schaue*	Behold the Sun
	Um Mitternächtige Stunde.	At the Midnight hour!
	Mit Steinen baue	In the lifeless ground
	Im leblosen Grunde.	Build thy rocky bower!
Back-ward	*So finde im Niedergang*	So, when in depths thou mourn,
	Und in des Todes Nacht	Find thou in Death's dark night
Stand	*Der Schöpfung neuen Anfang,*	Creation's pulse new-born
	Des Morgens junge Macht.	With living morning light.
	Die Höhen lass offenbaren	The Powers on high make known
For-ward	*Der Götter ewiges Wort;*	The eternal Word divine;
Quiet	*Die Tiefen sollen bewahren*	The Deeps must guard their own
	Den friedvollen Hort.	Peace, in their sacred shrine.
	Im Dunkel lebend	In gloom thou livest
	Erschaffe eine Sonne.	Create anew a Sun!
	Im Stoffe webend	In matter weavest –
For-ward	*Erkenne Geistes Wonne.*	Know Spirit-bliss begun!

Alongside the last four lines I wrote: *Dionysian*
With delight
legs crossed in E
(as in 'gate')
arms above in O

During one rehearsal that he watched, Steiner asked about the line *'The Deeps must guard their own'*.

'Why do you do this line downwards?'

'Because the depths are mentioned,' I answered.

'You do not have to do these lines downwards,' he said. 'The depths lie here above. In the world beyond the threshold you cannot speak of spatial relationships. The world where the true I is, is outside of space.'[11]

The following lines in Steiner's 'Dance of the Planets' should also be considered in this regard:

Es blauet der Himmel	The heavens become blue
Was sendet die Tiefe	What do the depths send
Aus Fernen zur Ende	From far distances to earth
Geheimnisvoll her?	Mysteriously?[12]

I only received the beautiful, complicated form for the verse 'Behold the sun...' from Rudolf Steiner years later.

The Whitsun verse: 'Where outer senses' knowledge ends...'

Shortly before Whitsun 1915, I asked Rudolf Steiner if he would agree to my doing the verse he gave at the end of his Whitsun lecture in Hamburg on May 15, 1910, as an introduction to his 1915 lecture. This was the only Whitsun verse we knew. Before this verse come the closing thoughts of the lecture:

> We can feel the thought of peace, of love, of harmony, which lies in the Whitsun thought ... We can feel it as an assurance of our hope for freedom and eternity ... And in the Whitsun thought we truly realise the power of those primal words which initiate after initiate passed on, and which reveal to us the meaning of wisdom and

eternity. These words, handed on from epoch to epoch, reveal to us the Whitsun thought; today for the first time they can sound forth exoterically, so that all humanity may understand them.

Being ranks with being in the widths of space,
Being follows being in the rounds of time.
Linger, Oh Man, in the widths of space, in rounds of time,

> Wo Sinneswissen endet
> Da stehet erst die Pforte,
> Die Lebenswirklichkeiten
> Dem Seelensein eröffnet;
> Den Schlüssel schafft die Seele,
> Wenn sie in sich erstarket
> Im Kampf, den Welten-mächte
> Auf ihrem eignen Grunde
> Mit Menschenkräften führen;
> Wenn sie durch sich vertreibet
> Den Schlaf, der Wissenskräfte
> An ihren Sinnesgrenzen
> Mit geistes-Nacht umhüllet. —

Whitsun verse 'Where outer senses' knowledge ends...', written by Rudolf Steiner in 1915.

You are in realms that fade and pass away.
Yet mightily your soul rises above them
When you divine or knowingly behold the eternal
Beyond the confines of space, beyond the flow of time.[13]

Steiner replied that he would like me to do not this verse, but a new Whitsun verse that he would give me. He went into his studio and, after a few minutes, brought me a sheet of paper on which he had written down the verse, 'Where outer senses' knowledge ends...' He said I should work on this and perform it before his Whitsun lecture. He did not give me a form for it or make any suggestions. I took the sheet to Marie Steiner and we set to work immediately.

The verse was first performed at Whitsun on May 22, 1915 in Dornach. In his lecture, which was called 'Pentecost Mood: Faust's Initiation with the Spirits of the Earth', Steiner spoke about a new element that would enter human consciousness through this verse. What differentiates this Whitsun verse from the one given in 1910 is the motif of the battle that is waged deep in the foundations of the human soul, something that was lacking in the previous verse. In the lecture Steiner says:

> This *Faust* is a perfect example of how complicated things really are in the depths of human nature. Something living in those depths is continually being exposed to the Ahrimanic-Luciferic powers of the world, but something else is living there as well that can be found by every human being who gives him- or herself over to the guidance of the Christ-impulse ... Why do we speak about a Guardian of the Threshold? Because it really is the case that what is rumbling and fighting and waging war in our everyday life in the very depths of the human soul was at first withdrawn from the human soul as though by an act of grace on

the part of the wisdom-filled guidance of the world.
Life goes on as if on a sort of surface, while all that
rumbling and fighting and warring are going on down
below. But even the life we experience on a daily basis
is a continual victory. It is just that this victory has to
be achieved over and over again.[14]

Earlier in the lecture, alluding to the new element mentioned above, he had said:

> Christ-knowledge is only possible when the human
> soul has a clear idea of the relationship of the
> Christ-impulse to the Luciferic and Ahrimanic
> forces. This is why the proclamation if the Luciferic
> and Ahrimanic aspect of the world is such an
> important part of what our spiritual-scientific
> movement had to take on, since it knew that it
> had to establish itself on the firm foundation of
> the Christ-impulse ... I think it is extraordinarily
> important for the human soul to feel that spiritual
> science has the task of bringing something
> absolutely new to people's awareness.[15]

The closing words of the lecture are:

> Today, however, I would like to close with this
> Pentecost verse, which expresses the essence of the
> ever-living, innermost nerve of our spiritual science,
> to which we have directed our attention today.[16]

Scenes from Faust, 1915

The great event of 1915 was the performances of scenes from *Faust*. On April 4, the scene in Faust's study on Easter night was performed with a change of scenery: black curtains were replaced by red before the song 'Christ is arisen'. Children also took part in the group of angels. The Spirit of the Earth was performed in the same way as is done today: behind a big billowing red curtain brought into movement by the artificially lengthened arms of the performer. In place of the head, Rudolf Steiner placed a shield, a big pentagram made with a few strokes to indicate eyes and nose.

On May 22, the Ariel scene was first performed on the stage in the Carpenter's Shop, with pale mauve curtains decorated with white and pink flowers. The elves (eight in all) were performed in eurythmy by children. They surrounded Ariel, standing on a small riser, and as indicated by Rudolf Steiner, at the words 'Then the little elves, great-souled / Haste to help, if help they can', descended and gathered around the sleeping Faust who was lying in the middle of the stage. This is how it was originally done on the big stage in the Goetheanum. Later on the children were replaced by adult eurythmists, and ultimately only two of these. The big semi-circular, three-tiered riser was lost to the flames that destroyed the Goetheanum on New Year's Eve 1923.

The first forms we received from Steiner were for the four groups of beings who accompany Ariel, the 'Watches' (*Faust: Part Two*, Act 1). The four forms were done by four groups of adult eurythmists, creating two curves to right and left. They are the same that are still done now. All eurythmy schools have a photocopy of these four forms (see diagram, p. 51).

By now, the eurythmy room in the south wing of the Goetheanum was finished. Rudolf and Marie Steiner often came up to work with us as we prepared for *Faust* and other performances.

The Ariel scene

Costumes

The group of elves around Ariel wore rose-coloured dresses. The remaining elves later wore the same as Ariel.

	Dress	*Veil*
Ariel (and the two accompanying elves):	White	Yellow
Group for First Watch (Gateway):	Green (bluish)	Mauve (reddish-purple)
Group for Second Watch (Moon):	Light blue	Yellow
Group for Third Watch (Seeds):	Green (yellowish)	Delicate reddish
Group for Fourth Watch (Sunrise):	(Steel) Blue	Red

When the curtain opens, Faust lies sleeping in the middle of the stage. He stirs restlessly. With the start of the musical introduction, Ariel appears and performs the gesture for *I*. Two accompanying elves waft in and perform the gesture for *E*. Together they form Group I. The four groups of Watches then appear one after another from right and left.

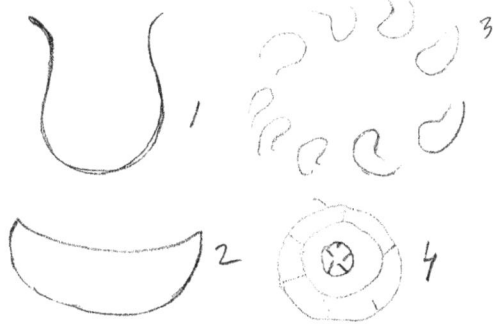

The sequence of the spatial forms, as drawn by Rudolf Steiner, for the four Watches that accompany Ariel in Faust: Part Two, Act 1.

Group II (First Watch) performing *O* gesture; does *AEIOU*
Group III (Second Watch) performing *A* gesture; does *AEIOU*
Group IV (Third Watch) performing *U* gesture; does *AEIOU*
Group V (Fourth Watch) performing *I* gesture; does *AEIOU*

When the petals, like sweet rain, / the middle group strong
Deck the earth with fluttering / the others weak
  spring,

When the fields are green again, / the middle group weak
And to men their blessing bring, / the others strong

Then the little elves, great- / the middle ones very weak
  souled,
Haste to help, if help they can, / the others weak

Saint or sinner, for they hold, / all make lively movements
Heart's compassion for each
  luckless man.[17]

During these lines, Faust makes a few restless movements.

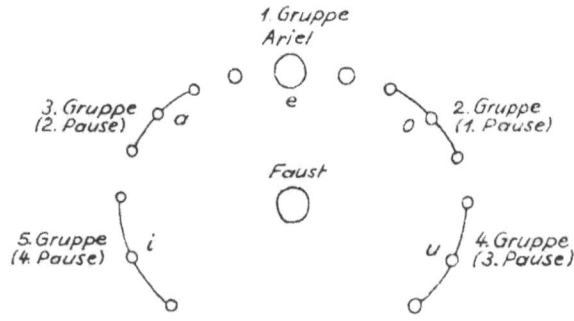

When Ariel says, 'You who surround his head...', Group I remains standing, while the other four groups form a circle around Faust, passing by each other.

1913–15: BUILDING UP

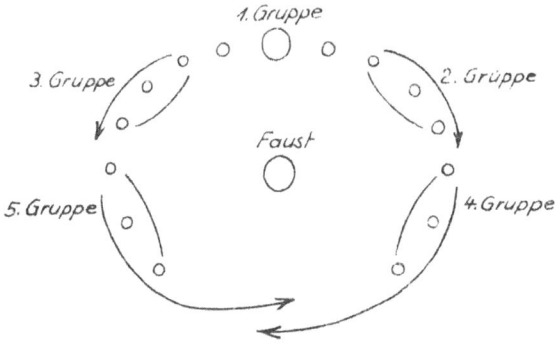

With 'Show now the noble elfin power,' all suddenly stop moving and stand in their original places.

With 'Soothe now the tumult ... of horrors past', all stand except the two elves from Group I who do the form from the introduction, and with the word 'horrors' make a sudden movement backwards.

From 'And, in the night's four vigils ...' until '... pity can impart', all stand.

With 'Pillow his head upon the sweet cool lawn', Group II (First Watch) moves towards Faust with the form from the introduction, bending deeply.

With 'Then bathe him in the dew from Lethe's flood', Group III (Second Watch) moves towards Faust with the form from the introduction, bending far back with the upper body. Group II (First Watch) moves away at the same time.

With 'Soon the cramp-stricken frame will lissom be / With strength renewed, through sleep, to meet the dawn', Group IV (Third Watch) moves towards Faust in a lively manner while the other groups stay calm. They make their gestures very low with 'cramp-stricken'.

With 'Fulfil, O elves, your lovely task aright', Group V (Fourth Watch) comes towards Faust with their gaze lifted up, as though they were seeing the sun.

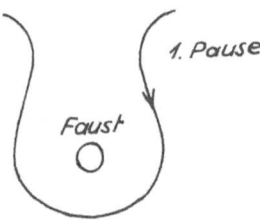

Then comes the music for Group II (First Watch) performing the *O* gesture. The form is made as they move around Faust forwards and backwards. Then with 'When cool airs...' the form is performed again but this time only forwards. Delicately and bending low with 'Closes soft the gates'.

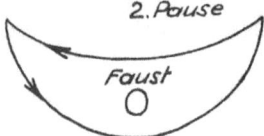

Music follows for Group III (Second Watch) performing the *A* gesture.

Then the line, 'Deep the falling of the night'. Very ceremonious; the sound gestures always above; upper body far backwards with the last lines. The arms never down, always remaining up. With fingers only: 'small sparks'; with arms quiet and only making movements with the fingers: 'glitter near' and 'shine afar'; with one arm down: 'mirrored in the lake'.

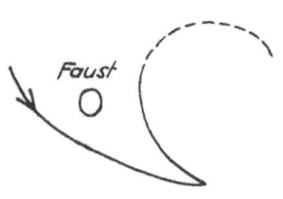

1913–15: BUILDING UP

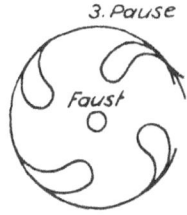

Music follows for Group IV (Third Watch) performing the *U* gesture. Then the text: 'Now the heavy hours have vanished'. Everything very lively with the arms in front of the chest.

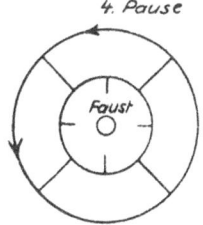

Music follows for Group V (Fourth Watch) preforming the *I* gesture. Then the text: 'Rise to wish...' Very decisive movements; lots of muscle tension in the arms downwards.

Sunrise is accompanied by a deafening noise. All the elves do a gesture of shock and self-protection. After the thunder all is very lively, beginning low and ending above, from 'Hark!' to 'Lest deafness comes'.

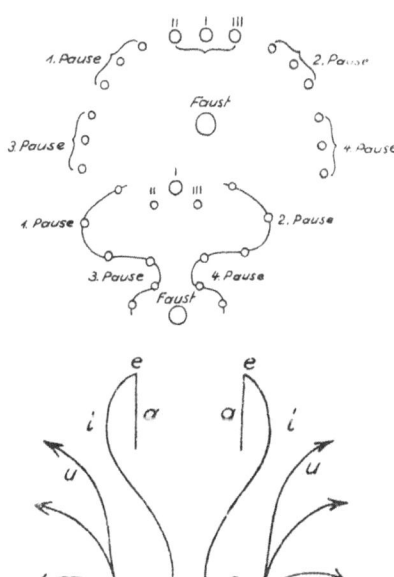

Ariel performs vowels, the others react with a few sounds. The following gestures are then performed on the following lines:

- 'new day': one step forwards, then backwards.
- 'grind': everyone takes a step to the side.
- 'thunder': a jump.
- 'Light': looking up; all with *I*-gesture down.
- 'trumpet': jump.
- 'trombone': jump even stronger.

- 'Sounds unheard': step backwards.
- 'Glide away to petalled bell': all withdraw in an in-winding spiral into the background of the stage and crouch (with the word 'deaf') around the Ariel group in the gesture of *B* (protecting oneself).

Then music; the elves remain immovable. At the end of the music, Faust stands up (who until then has only made small restless movements); at the same time, the elves move with him. Groups II, III, IV, V go back to their places in a spiral form with *A, E, I, O, U*. Every elf performs these vowels.

Faust's monologue

The elves accompany Faust's words with a few sounds: at the beginning of the speech, the rhyme of every second line is done with a slow movement, then later on the rhymed vowel in every line.

With the words, 'Send us to earth: to veil our troubled state,' the elves form a semicircle in front of Faust, coming from right and left. With the words, 'See the rainbow rising from this rage,' they divide in the middle and withdraw again to right and left. At the end, the elves group themselves at the front of the stage in front of Faust.

During the monologue:

- '... with pulses beating': lively gestures.
- '... the misty shapes': hands downwards.
- 'Look up on high!': right arm up, left down.

The last grouping with the music of the postlude:

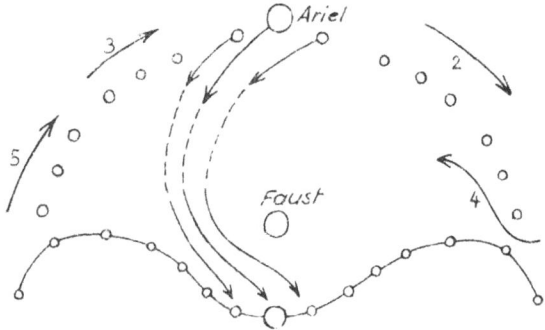

For the closing music, the following form is done in two rows. Ariel and the two accompanying elves do the form through the middle. All the elves, and also Ariel, do the vowels *A, E, I, O, U*; with the sound *I* all bend down low and then come up again and with a quick tempo resume their way. With the finishing position given above, all do a *U* gesture, upwards.

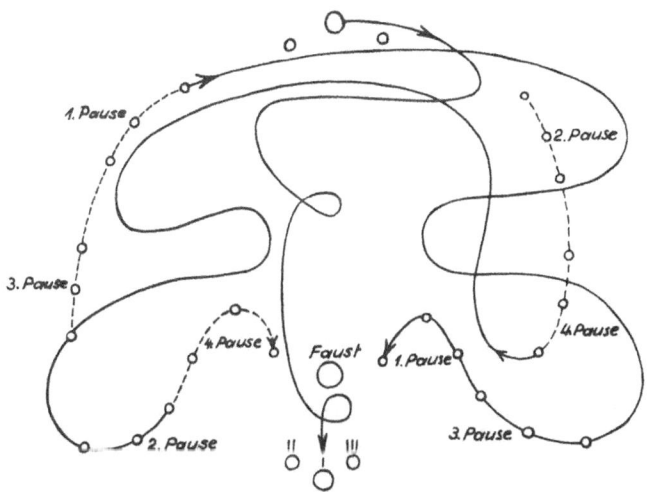

As already mentioned, the Ariel scene was first performed on May 22, 1915. Mieta Pyle-Waller played Faust. Jan Stuten conducted the orchestra, playing accompanying music that he had composed. In 1924 the scene was performed for the first time outside Dornach. The Stadttheater in Bern invited the group to give a public performance, and the part of Faust was played by the actor Edwin Froböse. At the dress rehearsal before the tour, Rudolf Steiner spoke the whole monologue with all the gestures, standing in the midst of the eurythmists doing the elves on the stage in the Carpenter's Shop. Then the scene was repeated with Edwin Froböse. In Bern the orchestra belonging to the theatre played the music composed by Jan Stuten for the Ariel scene. The text, apart from Faust's monologue, was spoken by Marie Steiner. Following this performance we repeated it in the Zürich Stadttheater. A year later the same program was performed in various places in Germany.

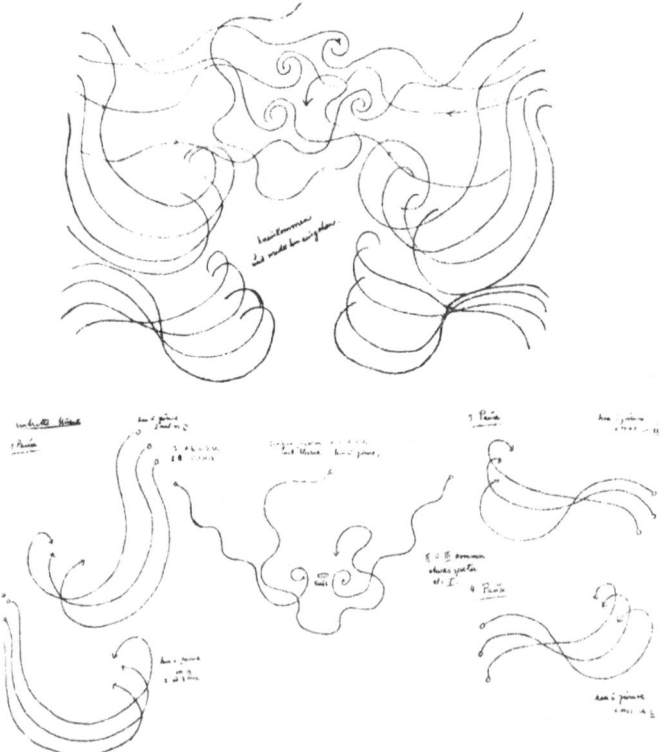

Facsimile of the drawing for the entrance (prelude). Rudolf Steiner provided this later on in addition.

Faust's Ascension, Prologue in Heaven, At Midnight

On August 15, 1915 'Faust's Ascension' was performed with all parts done in eurythmy, except those of Doctor Marianus and Mater Gloriosa. (The performance of this scene, done entirely in speech, was only possible later on, once Marie Steiner had trained her acting troupe.) There were two choruses of eurythmists on the stage: the chorus of anchorites and the echo, the first in yellow costumes, the second in purple. In the voluminous, dense veil of Pater Seraphicus, eight children were concealed, nestled close to him. Later, when Pater Seraphicus opened his veil, the children appeared and surrounded him with the words, 'Father, tell us as we wander...' in eurythmy. During the next part, the whole group ascended and led a heavenly dance around Pater Seraphicus at the top, forming into groups right and left like two clouds.

On August 19, the 'Prologue in Heaven' was also performed. For this scene costumes were sewn in three colours, with wings for the angels and also costumes with stoles for the archangels, all according to Rudolf Steiner's indications. The angels and archangels performed eurythmy. Marie Steiner recited for the heavenly hosts. God the Father and Mephistopheles recited their parts: the Lord invisible behind the stage, Mephistopheles in front on the proscenium. A challenging task was given to the eurythmist who was to perform the role of the archangel Michael: they would have to do all of the sounds, the vowels as well as the consonants, in eurythmy, while at the same time differentiating every word with Apollonian forms. In spite of the quick tempo and the great many movements, on no account was it allowed to appear hurried.

Joan Abels, a promising artistic eurythmist, was the first to take on the part, and she performed it exceedingly well. The audience could really sense the rivalling, ravaging storms with their 'tempestuous majesty', but also, in spite of this mighty appearance, something of the ruling harmony too.

The group of Michaelic angels accompanied the movements of the archangel Michael, some performing all of the vowels, the others all of the consonants.

Rudolf Steiner once said, while speaking of this scene, that Mephistopheles could also present what he has to say in eurythmy, but that unfortunately the devil's eurythmy had not yet been discovered. For this reason it would have to be done in materialistic mime. The angels and archangels had to accompany Mephistopheles' words with vowels that did not correspond, *O* for *E*, *U* and *Ü* for *A* and vice versa. Later on it was fixed as *A* = *Ü*; *E* = *O*; *I* = *U*; *O* = *E*; *U* = *I*; *Ü* = *A*; *Ö* = *EI*; other vowels with umlaut = *Ö*.

Soon afterwards, the scene 'At Midnight' (*Faust: Part Two*) was performed, with the women playing the four grey hags performing eurythmy.

In his introductory words to the performance of the 'Prologue in Heaven' in 1921, Steiner said that eurythmy lends itself very well to dramatic art in which the soul is lifted up to the supersensible; naturalistic stagecraft is inadequate for bringing the supersensible to the stage. Unfortunately, later indications by Steiner were partially ignored, with poor results despite the greater skill of the performers. In 1932, Marie Steiner called me from Paris to Dornach to work on scenes with eurythmists that had not been done under Steiner's direction. Fortunately, the most important indications for the other scenes, the ones for 'Walpurgis Night' (*Faust: Part One*) and 'At Midnight' (*Faust: Part Two*), had been preserved. The other *Faust* scenes for which Steiner had given indications will be described later (see p. 90).

Rudolf Steiner as actor

Although Rudolf Steiner never acted in performances, and for the most part during rehearsals only indicated the type of movements he wanted us to make without doing the gestures himself, he would sometimes demonstrate certain roles.

I have already mentioned how he characterised the gnomes during rehearsals in 1913 for the sylph and gnome dance in *The Soul's Awakening*. During our rehearsals for Faust in the Carpenter's Shop, he demonstrated a number of roles. His portrayal of Faust, especially in the scenes with the four grey women and with Worry, made a shattering impression on those of us who saw it. As a dramatic actor, Steiner was the same man of greatness, surpassing all others, as in his role of spiritual investigator and communicator of spiritual truths.

One demonstration I will never forget was his portrayal of the lemurs in the Burial Scene, where the angels and devils battle for Faust's eternal being. We were having difficulty grasping Steiner's directions and so he came onto the stage to show us what he meant. He took on a hunched posture and his arms and legs began to tremble, dangle, and flap about. The look in his eyes became dull, as though the light in them had been extinguished. Here, as when he demonstrated the gnomes, there was nothing of Steiner to be seen. Instead, a disintegrating remnant of a human being stood before our astonished eyes. In the next moment he took on his own form again and in a friendly manner said, 'Yes, that is how the lemurs really are.'

Steiner also demonstrated many of the roles in the Christmas plays. Once in a rehearsal he portrayed Joseph as ancient and looking around a little stupidly. He came to the front of the stage, leaning on a long stick. Suddenly he stumbled, intentionally, and fell on his face with open mouth and wide-open eyes looking at the audience. 'This is the way Joseph was played in earlier times,' he said, getting up from the floor. 'He was experienced as a kind of fool or idiot.' He later remarked that, artistically speaking, it was more interesting to play the part of an idiot, and that he personally would much rather take on that role than the role of the main hero.

Pater Noster and the Gospel of John

The next forms that were given by Rudolf Steiner were the drawings for the Lord's Prayer. I already had forms for the first part from the time I had worked with Marie Steiner in Villa Hansi. Steiner drew this original form in my notebook. Of all his eurythmy forms, this is the only one of its kind with a specific line or a little form for nearly every word.

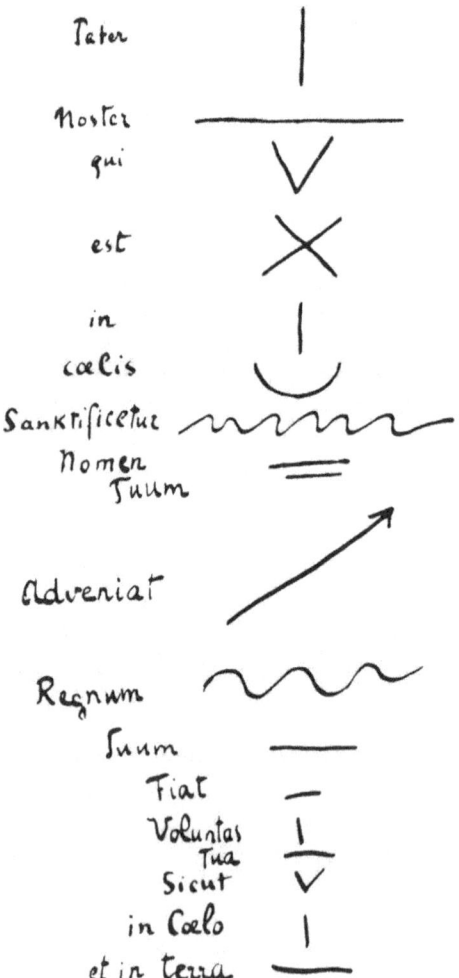

He wanted this prayer to be done in eurythmy in Latin. He recited it, very slowly, and I had to do it entirely *with vowels*. In the course of working, he pointed out that I should do 'big gestures only for the emphasised vowels.' That was the only time Steiner gave the indication to do purely vowels. I understood this indication for the Lord's Prayer to be an exception. For the second part of the prayer, I did not need to only do the emphasised vowels.

From a copy of the original, reduced to half the size.

Steiner also gave the zones and directions: *'sanctificetur Nomen Tuum'* / 'Hallowed be Thy Name' – above the head; *'adveniat regnum Tuum'* / 'Thy Kingdom Come' – in the middle; *'fiat voluntas Tua'* / 'Thy will be done' – arms down, head turned to the right.

He gave no forms for the second part of the prayer, after 'On Earth as it is in Heaven'. He said that I could do them myself, only giving the following instruction: instead of *'panem nostrum quotidianum'*, for 'our daily bread' I should use *'panem nostrum supersubstantialem'*.* For the last words, *'libera nos a malo'* / 'Deliver us from evil', I was to perform *'a malo'* / 'evil', with a big *A* – arms stretched downwards behind the back and the palms of the hands facing outwards. Then, after a pause, the word 'Amen' with stretched arms in *A* up above the head (directed somewhat forwards), with no *E* added, but ending with the *A* gesture.

The *Pater Noster*, with the above indications in Latin, was only performed once during Rudolf Steiner's lifetime, at the Christmas celebration in Basel on December 22, 1918. It was done in front of the Christmas tree in the room of the Branch of the Anthroposophical Society. Marie Steiner had chosen the texts and recited them: the *Pater Noster*, then the annunciation of the angels to the shepherds from the Gospel of St. Luke in German, and at the end a prayer in an old Slavic language. Rudolf Steiner wanted eurythmy to be done in various languages.

In his lifetime, the beginning of the Gospel of St. John ('In the beginning was the Word...') was never performed. He expressly did not want this. That is why there are no forms or indications for this. I have kept to this, also in teaching. It seems right to me even now to keep one's distance and not

---

* Both *quotidianum* and *supersubstantialem* are translations of the Greek, *epiousios* (ἐπιούσιος), found in Matt 6:11 and Luke 11:3. Although traditionally translated as 'daily', a more literal translation of *epiousios* might be 'supersubstantial', referring to something that is essential for life. It isn't clear why Steiner insisted on this latter translation, although it's possible he had a more spiritual form of sustenance in mind besides earthly bread.

try to do it in eurythmy because our present ability to form it is still insufficient.

The Portal of Inititation, scene 7: Devachan

It wasn't long before Rudolf Steiner's lectures were preceded by artistic presentations of two or three items of eurythmy, with Marie Steiner reciting any text or verses. Steiner disapproved of purely musical introductions to his lectures. We can gauge the significance eurythmy had for him by the remarks he made a year later following a Sunday afternoon eurythmy performance for members of the Anthroposophical Society. The performance was very poorly attended and that evening he began his lecture with approximately the following words: 'At the eurythmy performance this afternoon most of you shone by your absence. You must know that if you do not participate in eurythmy, either actively on the stage or as members of the audience, then I do not need to hold any more lectures because you will not be able to take in what I have to say and I will have spoken in vain.'

In the production or enjoyment of art, human beings in the present make the connection between what they were in pre-earthly life and what they will be in the life after death.

> But in art ... we can take a step back from life and a few steps nearer to what we were in pre-birth life and what we will be in life after death ... in art we can call into the present moment – as far as this is possible for us in our physical state – what connects us with the spirit. You see, art acquires its distinctive luminosity by transposing us, albeit naively, into the immediate presence of the world of the spirit.[18]

One of the first performances in eurythmy was the first part of scene 7 from the Mystery Drama, *The Portal of Initiation*.[19]

Marie Steiner recited the words of Maria, standing on the stage dressed in yellow. I did the soul forces in eurythmy, beginning with Philia, then changing the veil quickly behind the stage to reappear as Astrid, before changing the veil again and reappearing as Luna. I repeated the transformation after Maria's second speech. Louise Clason and Käthe Milscher, the original performers of the soul forces Astrid and Luna in the Mystery Dramas in Munich, recited for the eurythmy. These three veils, light green for Philia, light crimson for Astrid, and purple for Luna, were the very first veils in Dornach. I bought them shortly beforehand (by chance, as one says) in a sale in Basel, the colours happening to be just the colours that corresponded to the soul forces.

Our wardrobe was very primitive in those first years. We did not have the means to buy coloured silk dresses, and instead dyed a few simple cotton dresses in various colours. Then, in 1921, the eurythmy wardrobe was enlarged. One day Marie Steiner informed us with delight that Rudolf Steiner had received a letter, together with a small amount of money, from a young girl belonging to an anthroposophical family in Stuttgart. Ruth Unger-Palmer had heard him speak on a visit to her town about how poorly the eurythmists were dressed, and she had suggested to her friend that the money they had saved together, money they usually spent on books each year, be sent to Steiner in Dornach instead. The decision was thus taken to buy veils to replace those few we possessed and which were pretty worn out. Soon afterwards, during a performance, our Dornach friends were pleased to see the large new veils in seven colours, which we wore over our former white dresses. There was not enough money to purchase coloured dresses, which is probably why only the colour of the veils is mentioned in the early descriptions of forms and nothing about dresses.

I would now like to describe Steiner's indications for this scene, on which the performances were based for a long time. His further indications point towards future developments.

Costumes

According to Rudolf Steiner's indications, the dresses should be the following, which differs from the above description:

	Dress	Veil
Maria:	light-mauve	light-mauve
Philia:	deepest rose	green shot with red
Astrid:	white	white
Luna:	rose	light-blue shot with rose

Luna chorus:
1: orange
2: blue
3 and 4: purple

Astrid chorus:
1: blue – purple
2 and 3: light-red
4: yellow

Philia chorus:
1: light-blue
2: yellow
3 and 4: mauve

This is one way to perform the scene:

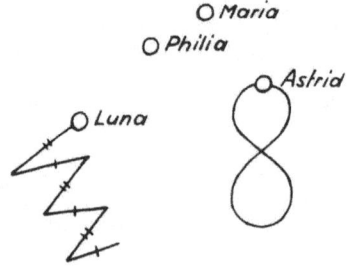

Maria recites or performs the vowels for her part while standing.

The three soul forces proceed as follows. While standing:
- Philia: holding *I* up;
- Astrid: *A* in the middle;
- Luna: *U* down.

For the text:
- Philia: standing, does all vowels in the zone above;
- Astrid: moves with iambic rhythm in a lemniscate, doing consonants in the middle zone;
- Luna: moves rhythmically in amphimacer-spondee in the form shown (left), doing consonants and vowels downward.

Rudolf Steiner also gave indications for a second way to do the spatial forms with the Mercury Prelude. He gave these during the course in 1915. Leopold van der Pals composed the music. As the drawing below shows, the form is simplified in comparison to the planetary seal. In this instance, the Mercury Prelude is like a message from the spiritual world.

The main performers do as follows:

- Maria does the indicated Apollonian forms. She does only *I*, *U* (also *AU*), *A* (expressing 'call', 'longing', and 'knowledge-communication'), without reciting. She does concrete and abstract noun forms, as well as verb forms in space.
- Philia does vowel gestures (done as high above as possible). Her chorus does consonants.
- Astrid weaves consonants and vowels into one another in the space in front of her. Her chorus does the same, having prior to this decided together which consonants she leaves to them. Luna does consonants in the lower zone and her chorus the vowels.

Other scenes can be done in this way. For instance, scenes from plays by Sophocles and Aeschylus, or from the *Bride of*

Messina; also Goethe's poems for the Festival Plays – that is, in pieces performed around a central person, the central figure or figures can do as Maria does.

Simplified Mercury Prelude

When the music begins Philia enters (with *I* up), followed by Astrid (with *A* in front), Luna (with *U* down) and then Maria (in *E* gesture with arms crossed on the chest, building up *I*, *A*, *U* as she moves). At the crescendo, the choruses appear from three sides, each one consisting of between four to six people, and form a semi-circle around the main characters who continue in their form until the end of the music.

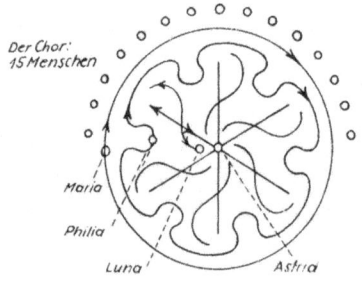

In order to reach the starting positions for the text, follow the transitions from the end positions of the Mercury Prelude, as shown in the dotted lines in the next drawing.

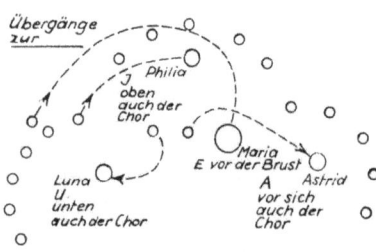

The stage can also be arranged on four levels, with Maria on the highest step and the three soul forces on the descending steps. However, this indication was never put into practice.

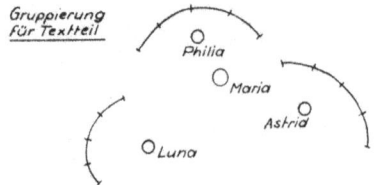

The sequence of the Devachan scene, line-by-line, is as follows. Maria only does *I, A, U* to each of her lines.

Line:	Maria:	Soul forces:
1	Call (soul gesture) *I*	During Maria's speech, from 'You my sisters...'
2	Call *I*	until '...for soaring flight' (line 22),
3	Call *I*	the soul forces do the following:
4	Longing *U*	
5	Longing *U*	Philia stands with *I* up.
6	Knowledge *A*	
7	Knowledge *A*	Astrid, with *A* in front.
8	Knowledge *A*	
9	Communication *A*	Luna, with *U* down.
10	Communication *A*	
11	Call *I*	Philia's chorus does consonants up.
12	Call *I*	
13	Longing *U* (like *AU*)	Astrid's chorus is divided:
14	Longing *U* (like *AU*)	vowels and consonants in front
15	Longing *U* (like *AU*)	(until line 22).
16	Communication *A*	Luna's chorus does vowels down.
17	Communication *A*	
18	Communication *A*	
19	Communication *A*	
20	Longing *U*	Astrid's chorus is divided:
21	Longing *U*	vowels and consonants in
22	Longing *U*	front (until line 22).

Turns to Philia:

23–29	Call *I* up	From 'And so, my Philia...' until '...dances of the Spheres' (line 32).
30	Call *I* up	Philia standing, with vowels up; chorus in *I*.
31	*A* up	Astrid – *A*; chorus does agreed-upon sounds.
32	*A* up	Luna – *U*; chorus – vowels.

Turns to Astrid:

33–39	Call *I* in front	'And you too, Astrid...'
40	Call *I* with other arm	Astrid vowels and a few consonants.
41	*A* Communication	Chorus in *A*.
42	*A* Communication	Philia – *I*; chorus – consonants. Luna – *U*; chorus – vowels.

Line:	Maria:	Soul forces:
	Turns to Luna:	
43–	Call *I* down	From 'And you, O sturdy
47		Luna...' until '...to the seeker.' (line 50).
48	Call *I* down	Luna standing consonants; chorus *U*.
49	*A* down	Astrid – *A*; chorus – mixed sounds.
50	*A* down	Philia – *I*; chorus – consonants.

Philia brings it all together as a response, performing the vowels above as well as the forms.

Lines 51–58:
From 'I will imbue myself...'   'Fulfilment' towards Maria – up;
to '...may reach your goal.'   chorus in *I*.
                                Astrid – *A*; chorus – mixed sounds.
                                Luna – *U*; chorus – vowels.

Astrid then moves in 'fulfilment' and weaves together vowels and consonants.

Lines 59–67:
From 'And I will weave...'   'Fulfilment' towards Maria in
to '...the rays of soul.'   middle zone; chorus – *A*.
                                Philia – *I*; chorus – consonants.
                                Luna – *U*; chorus – vowels

Luna moves in 'fulfilment', weaving consonants.

Lines 68–76:
From 'I will enwarm...'   'Fulfilment' down; chorus *U*.
to '...certainty of knowledge.' Astrid – *A*; chorus – mixed sounds.
                                Philia – *I*; chorus – consonants.

Maria's response follows, broken down into three parts.

Lines 77–85:
From 'From Philia's horizons...' Maria – *A* up (no other sounds).
to '...the world's despair.'   Philia – *I*; chorus – vowels up.
                                Astrid – *A*; chorus – mixed sounds.
                                Luna – *U*; chorus – consonants.

Line: Maria: *Soul forces:*
Lines 86–94:
From 'From Astrid's weaving...'   Maria – *A*, a little lower.
to '...who are joy-entreating.'   Philia – *I*; chorus – vowels.
                                        Astrid – *A*; chorus – mixed sounds.
                                        Luna – *U*; chorus – consonants.

Lines 95–104:
From 'From Luna's strength...'   Maria – *A* right down.
to '...in world-life-breathing.'   Philia – *I*; chorus – vowels.
                                        Astrid – *A*; chorus – mixed sounds.
                                        Luna – *U*; chorus – consonants down.

Philia moves in 'fulfilment', performing vowels. Chorus performs consonants up in 'fulfilment'.

Lines 105–113:
'I will entreat...'   Astrid, with chorus in *A*.
to '... to heavenly heights.'   Luna, with chorus in *U*.

Astrid performs vowels and a few consonants with forms (discuss with chorus which consonants are left for them to do).

Lines 114–122:
From 'I will guide...'   Philia, with chorus in *I*.
to '...to sons of men.'   Luna, with chorus in *U*.

Luna performs consonants with forms; chorus performs vowels down with 'fulfilment'.

Lines 123–136:
From 'I will...'   Philia, with chorus in *I*.
to '...for all eternity.'   Astrid, with chorus in *A*.

Maria does *I* (up) during Philia's words and at the very end, during the last two lines, she does *A* (up); with Astrid's words *I* (in front, left arm towards Astrid) to *A* in front; with Luna's words *I* (down, right arm towards Luna) to *A* down. All three times *A* in 'fulfilment' the arms are carried from the front to the back.

Line: Maria:	Soul forces:
Lines 137–140:	
'With you, my sisters,	Maria does vowels (mainly *I* and *AU*) with forms.
united for this earnest work,	Philia – vowels; chorus – consonants.
I shall succeed	Astrid – mixed; chorus – mixed.
in what I long to do.'	Luna – consonants; chorus – vowels.

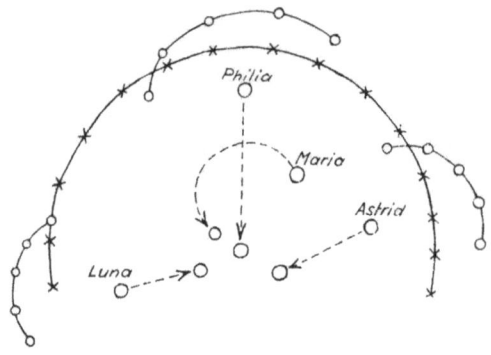

A silent regrouping then follows (indicated by the dotted lines in the drawing above) while the chorus members place themselves in a semicircle at the back, with the front arm more downward, the back arm higher toward each other like a protecting chain.

For the end positions, the main characters do the following gestures:
- Maria – left arm stretched over Philia's head, right arm in the middle position somewhat forwards toward Philia as though protecting;
- Luna in *U* towards Philia;
- Astrid in *A* towards Philia;
- Philia – right arm in *I* up.

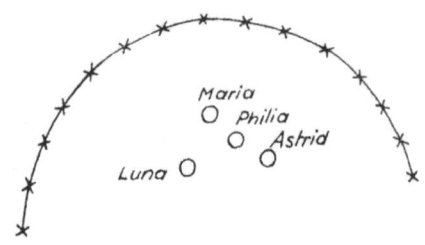

Rudolf Steiner also gave the following instructions for another way to do the scene:

Musical introduction: only music.
Singing (whether choir or solo or both, he did not say).

Recitation: without music, singing, or eurythmy.
Eurythmy: without accompaniment through recitation or music.
Recitation: again alone (the eurythmists withdraw).
Singing: again alone.
Musical *Nachtakt* or epilogue: again only music.

This version, which Steiner characterised as a more perfect or complete way to do it, was never performed during his lifetime nor until the time of this writing.* Steiner said that eurythmy without recitation or music corresponds to a certain degree of perfection, and that in the far future, after further development, eurythmy will no longer need accompaniment. Ideally, the text should be recited alone first so that the audience can connect themselves with the content of the poem. Only after that should the text be performed in eurythmy, accompanied by the recitation. The simultaneous experience of 'audible' and 'visible' speech is awkward as one can neither listen properly, nor connect oneself through looking with the eurythmy.

I would like to add two quotations, especially the second regarding the Mercury Prelude. Rudolf Steiner said in his introduction to a eurythmy performance on February 19, 1918 in Munich:

> Through this we are really led back to the principles of the early temple dance because all true temple art was intended to penetrate human life with the power of the word. But by 'word' was not understood what we understand by it, but rather it meant the wisdom sounding through the world

* The scene has since been performed according to these indications – *Trans.*

in the harmony of the spheres that is expressed in the most diverse realms. This is given a pure copy in human speech, a somewhat more abstract expression in human singing, and materialises in instrumental music. It can be redeemed when ... the whole human organism is brought into forming and movement.[20]

In the lecture he gave on April 21, 1924, in Dornach, Steiner speaks about those ancient mysteries – the Ephesian Mysteries in particular – in which the wisdom of the moon is not only taught but inwardly experienced:

> Because certain Moon-beings could gaze on Mars, we were enabled to organise within our etheric bodies *the capacity for speech*. Because these beings were able to gaze on Mercury, we acquired what enables us to construct within our etheric body *the aptitude for movement*.
>
> If people desire to speak in accordance with these Mysteries of the Moon at the present time, it is possible to give expression to them in an entirely different form: this can be done by eurythmy. Eurythmy develops of out speech. Having investigate the mysteries of language, by allowing the Moon-beings to instruct us in what they are able to observe when gazing on Mars, we make further investigations. We then notice how what we investigate changes, if after having directed our observation to Mars we direct it to Mercury. Thus when we turn from what the Moon-beings experience through Mars to what they experience with regard to Mercury, we pass from the human aptitude for the production of sound to the human aptitude for eurythmy. This is to explain the matter in its cosmic aspect.[21]

The Mystery Drama seals in eurythmy

According to Rudolf Steiner, the simplified Mercury Prelude is not only to be used as an introduction to the Devachan scene, but can also be used as a spiritual message in other dramatic works. Already in the eurythmy room of the first Goetheanum he mentioned using it in *Faust*, in the Prologue in Heaven, whereby the spatial forms of the soul forces Philia, Astrid and Luna could be done by the three archangels Raphael, Gabriel and Michael. Unfortunately, I did not ask, either then or later on, when we practised these scenes on the finished stage of the first Goetheanum, how to incorporate the voice of God eurythmically. Rudolf Steiner also said nothing about Maria's form. Could this be done with the twelve fixed stars?

In the completed first Goetheanum, Steiner made us aware that the seals for the four Mystery Dramas could also be done in eurythmy as an introduction to each play. I asked how one could do eurythmy for the seal for *The Portal of Initiation*, which has curved lines that open outwards. He replied that the seven eurythmists who were moving along these curves would need to move seven times behind the columns on the stage into what was for the audience the invisible world, as though entering another dimension. No mention was made of possible musical accompaniment. It was never done in eurythmy. As with so many other things, this remains a task for the future, which can hardly be done without Rudolf Steiner.

The first eurythmy teachers

Marie Steiner took charge of the eurythmy work. The rehearsals for the scenes to be performed took place in the Carpenter's Shop and also the performances for the members of the society. Children also took part.

From time to time eurythmists came from Germany, where they were working, to join in the performances, and when

Marie Steiner travelled in Germany she was able to work intensively with them. In the summer of 1915, we were joined by three teachers who greatly enriched our performances in Dornach, Elisabeth Dolfuss-Baumann, Lory Maier-Smits and Erna van Deventer-Wolfram. On Sundays, the newcomers performed poems they had worked on in Germany alongside presentations by local eurythmists showed, they also joined in with the group pieces.

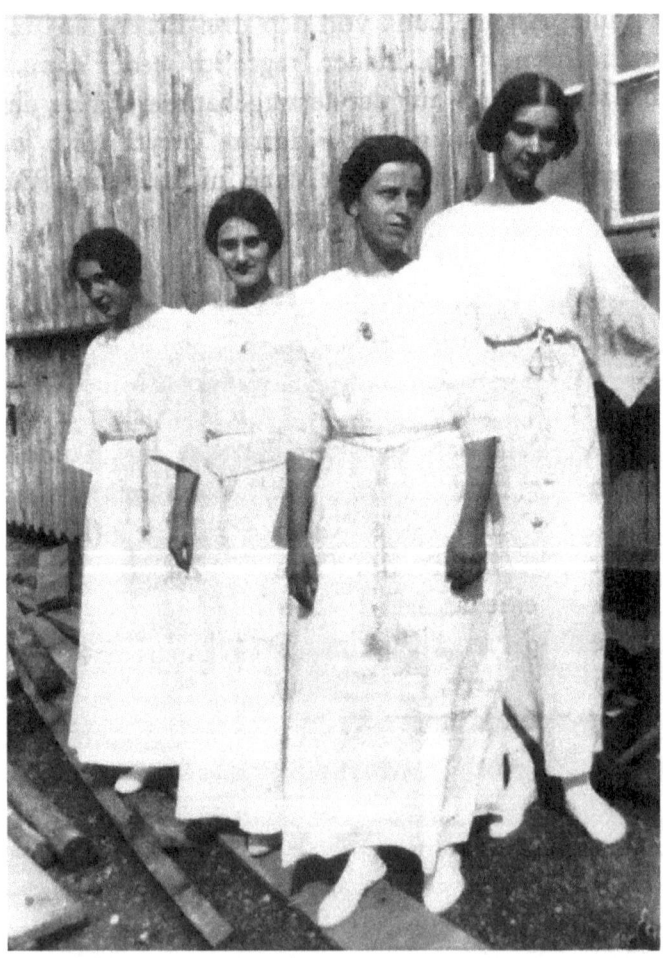

From left to right: Elisabeth Dollfuss-Baumann, Lory Maier-Smits, Erna van Deventer-Wolfram and Tatiana Kisseleff. Photograph taken during the eurythmy course in 1915.

1915–18: Expansion and Deepening

All that I have said so far about the early years of eurythmy belongs to the first phase of its development, which lasted exactly three years: from August 1912 to August 1915. A new phase began in August/September 1915, with a course in which the three eurythmy teachers who had joined us that summer, Lory Maier-Smits, Erna van Deventer-Wolfram and Elisabeth Dollfuss-Baumann, took part alongside myself and Marie Steiner. The three mothers of the eurythmy teachers also participated as did Mieta Pyle-Waller. Annemarie Dubach-Donath later described the course in wonderful detail in her book, *The Basic Principles of Eurythmy*, in which she also added her own work on the subject.

On that occasion Rudolf Steiner gave us the 'second chapter' of eurythmy, called Apollonian eurythmy. He began the course with the words:

> Until now we have been spelling; now we will take in the whole, which will make things more inward, by going over from the picture of the word into the picture of the meaning.[1]

Tone eurythmy

The first foundations of tone eurythmy were also given at that time. Rudolf Steiner said: 'The tone appears *through* the whole human being; the spoken word *on* the human being.' He then

he spoke about how to express the musical intervals. He drew on the blackboard and told us to do the following:

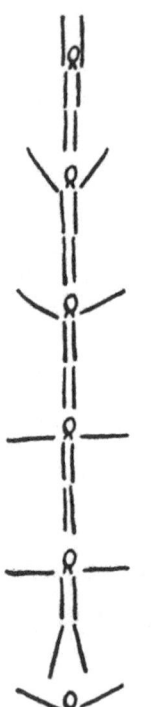

1. Arms lifted upwards parallel to one another, feet together: the prime interval.

2. Arms at an angle of 30°: the second interval.

3. Arms at an angle of 60°: the third interval.

4. Arms out at the side in the form of a cross: the fourth interval.

5. Feet apart at an angle: the fifth interval.

6. Arms at an angle of 60°, feet apart: the sixth interval.

7. Arms at an angle of 30°, feet apart: the seventh interval.

Steiner then spoke about the position of the arms and feet and the jumps forwards and backwards for the minor scale. He added a drawing in profile and let us practise this.

At the end of the course, we drew the tones of C major with differentiated spaces for the half tones between E and F and between B and C, showing them with small angles of 15°; we then did the same for the A minor scale. Afterwards, Steiner showed us how to perform the half tones, the sharps, and the flats by bending the elbows to create either a right angle or a rounded gesture. He also gave directions on how to present musical pieces in the form of a triangle: the person standing at the point of the triangle would sing, the one standing in front on the right would do the sounds, and the one standing in front on the left would do tones. In 1916 we made a few attempts at this. The first was with a performance of 'The Worm's Confession', the humoresque by Christian Morgenstern with music by Max Schuurman:

There lives inside a mussel
A worm so wondrously;
He has with gentle bustle
Revealed his heart to me.

It pounded never resting,
That aching little heart!
You think that I am jesting?
O don't think you're so smart.

There lives inside a mussel
A worm so wondrously;
He has with gentle bustle
Revealed his heart to me.[2]

Mieta Pyle-Waller sang, with two eurythmists standing with her in the triangle, one doing the speech sounds, the other the tones as Steiner had shown us. We rotated positions after the first and second verses. Other poems set to music were done in the same manner.

To begin with we practised tone eurythmy standing still, conscientiously doing every jump in the major and minor scales. But very soon we began to do primitive forms, which we drew ourselves. This first attempt to go from standing to moving forms took place about a year after being given the first indications in tone eurythmy. Along with a few other eurythmists I tried out a simple melody on a little symmetrical form drawn on the stage, replacing the standing jumps in the major scales with light, springing steps forward. We showed this attempt to Steiner who approved and gave the indication for moving forwards in minor: the earlier jump forwards and backwards was replaced by a pulling after or dragging of the foot, like the short in a trochee. We practised this way of moving, but in the performances we still did the tones standing still (as, for instance, in the performances of the sirens in the *Classical Walpurgis Night in Faust: Part Two*). The first musical forms were performed to '*Bist du bei mir*' ('If you are with me') from the Sacred Songs by Bach. Rudolf Steiner indicated that one of the three performers sing the song on the stage without doing eurythmy, while the others alternately move and do tone eurythmy.[3]

Rudolf Steiner said that performing eurythmy sounds accompanied by singing could only be done in exceptional cases. For instance, the message from the *Chemical Wedding of Christian Rosenkreutz* by Valentin Andreae, which begins with the words: 'Today, today is our Lord's wedding', was sung backstage. Meanwhile, onstage, the chorus moved in lemniscates as they performed tone eurythmy, while a second group standing at the front performed the vowels to the sung text. The chorus wore white dresses and yellow stoles, and the second group wore a red stole.

Tone eurythmy developed especially through Hendrika Hollenbach's work with children, for which she compiled systematic exercises along with little compositions. This formed the content of the courses in tone eurythmy. Hendrika Hollenbach also worked with many eurythmists in this field.

During this course we also received the so-called Preludes: Happy, Sad or Elegiac, Satirical, Cosmic, the *TIAOAIT*, as well as the Mercury Prelude for scene 7 of *The Portal of Initiation* (see p. 68). Rudolf Steiner pointed out that the Mercury Prelude, insofar as it presented a spiritual message, could also be done before other dramatic works. He gave the example of

1915–18: EXPANSION AND DEEPENING

the beginning of *Faust* tragedy and indicated that the forms given for Philia, Astrid, and Luna should instead be performed by the archangels in the 'Prologue in Heaven'.

At the end of this course four dances were given: two 'Dances of the Planets', 'The Twelve Moods' (see p. 117) and the satire 'The Song of Initiation'.

The round podium

During that course, from August to September 1915, Rudolf Steiner said that the progression of the octaves should be done on raised steps, which he intended to have built for tone eurythmy. This round podium would need to have several steps so that the musical scales could be clearly presented with the circle divided into twelve parts. The thirteenth tone would be done on the top step. Through this progression an upward spiral would thus appear. Steiner added that it was going to take a lot of practice for us to acquire the technique of jumping from one step to the other, especially to manage the jump backwards from a lower step to a higher one. The back should never be turned to the audience, and the jump must be done with ease and grace.

I drew this according to Rudolf Steiner's indications. The different octaves should be done on different steps, starting with the lowest octave on the lowest step (first tone C). The scale is to be done in such a way that the circle is divided into

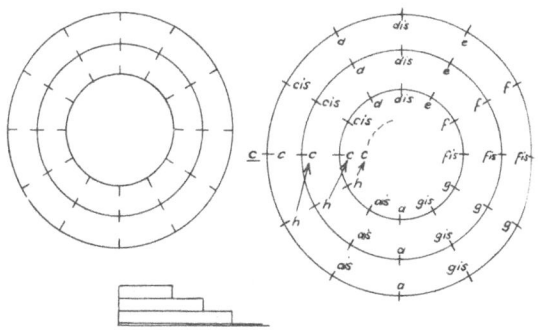

Diagram for the round podium for tone eurythmy (note: in German, Cis stands for C#).

twelve parts. Steiner said that the rests would be expressed by a step back. Unfortunately, the use of such a round podium was never attempted.

'The Song of Initiation'
Until 1920 only the indication for the paths of the planets and the changing of the order of the paths for Mercury and Venus had been given.

For the performance in the first Goetheanum in October 1920, Rudolf Steiner added that the figures of the zodiac, who were sitting on the floor, should rise only when the sun approaches them, languidly do their seven-line stanzas in eurythmy, and then sink back down into sleep. The sun should have a luciferic, unkempt red wig and wear a white dress with a dull yellow veil. At the end of each verse she is always a little behind and must each time run back to her proper place in agitation.

On one occasion, when we were working on the text for 'The Twelve Moods' and the satire 'The Song of Initiation', Steiner said that we should not think that the gods are always serious; they can laugh and do so very often. He added, smiling, that you could hear roaring laughter in heaven every time human beings behaved foolishly on earth.

Many other eurythmists participated in these last lessons. Steiner put us into groups and explained how we should move through the space. He and Marie Steiner recited the texts for the dances of the stars.

Steiner later wrote about this course:

> The instruction for the ensouled shaping of the speech forms was first given to the students in this room built into the south wing of the Goetheanum. The interior architecture of this space in particular was to be a eurythmy come to rest just as the eurythmy movements in it are moving sculptural forms out of the same spirit as the forms at rest.[4]

The White Room

The significance Rudolf Steiner gave to anthroposophists doing eurythmy can be measured by how important it was for him that eurythmy continue uninterrupted. One can see this from the arrangements made early on in the building of the first Goetheanum. After I had to stop my eurythmy lessons in the village pub in Dornach in the autumn of 1914, I continued with classes for adults in the Carpenter's Shop, and classes for children in the two rooms on the ground floor of the house in which Rudolf and Marie Steiner lived. One day Steiner told me that he and Marie Steiner would have to be away for a longer time than usual. He had given instructions that during this time the completion of the room for eurythmy – later known as the White Room – in the south wing of the building should have priority over all other work. The foreman of the work had been charged to hand over the keys to me as soon as the room was fit for use. I was delighted with this, and I asked whether I really was allowed to teach in the space before he had dedicated it. He answered that there was no need to wait, but to proceed without dedication.

'As soon as you have the key,' he said, 'you can begin working.'

During Rudolf and Marie Steiner's absence the room was indeed finished. The foreman joyfully handed me the key and confirmed that Rudolf Steiner had stressed that the room should be completed as soon as possible. That evening I informed the students that we would be moving into the room and the first lesson would be held there the following morning.

Our entrance into the room had a dramatic prelude. A few of the older members, who felt responsible for what happened in the Goetheanum and knew nothing about the arrangement regarding the room, felt it their duty to send the children away when they arrived. When I appeared at ten o'clock with my key, I too had to endure their reproaches. At this critical moment, Mieta Pyle-Waller appeared, and her testimony resolved the tension. She had personally heard from Rudolf Steiner about the arrangement before his departure, including the instruction about handing over the key. She confirmed my statements, and we were allowed into the room. I asked her to call back the students, who had not gone far.

In the years that followed, a great deal of eurythmy was enthusiastically practised in that room. After returning from a lecture tour, Rudolf and Marie Steiner often came to see the work we had been doing. Steiner would give us forms and indications, among the very first were those belonging to the four 'watches' from the Ariel scene in *Faust*. I also practised there on various poems, including some by Christian Morgenstern, which Marie Steiner sometimes recited for me. I showed a few of these to Rudolf Steiner who said that the eurythmy forms he had given us so far were not adequate for them; other forms and ways of expression would need to be found. We did not have to wait long either. During the second eurythmy course that took place August 18 to September 11, 1915, we received many new indications that enriched eurythmy immeasurably.[5]

Unfortunately, the photograph that was taken of the room does not adequately convey what it was like to enter this

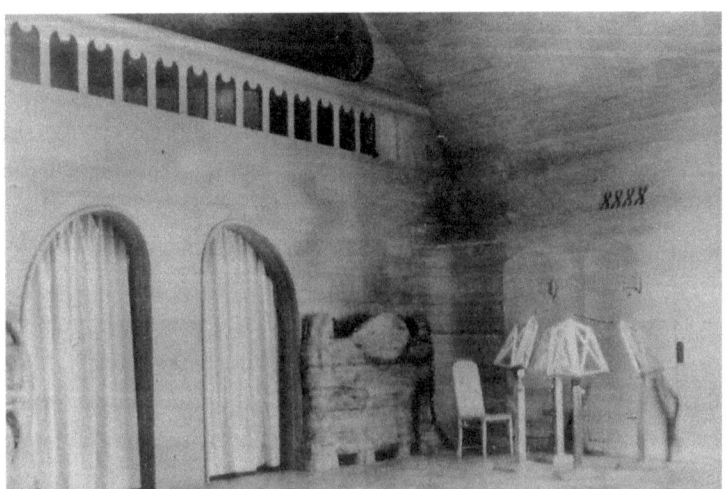

The White Room in the south wing of the first Goetheanum.

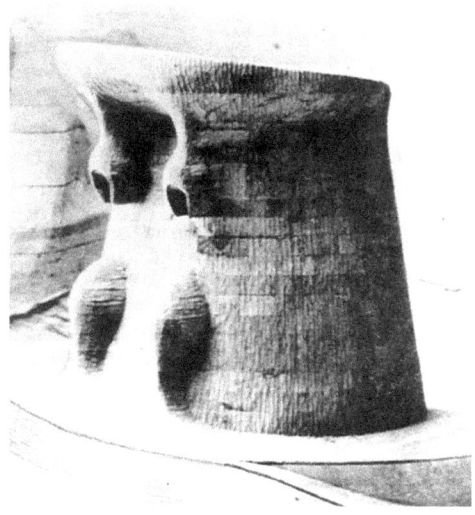

The speaker's lectern in the White Room.

unique space, to experience the beautiful architecture of this 'eurythmy come to rest'.[6] It also gives no idea of the effect it had on the children who worked in this room. All that remains physically perceptible of this space, which played such an important role in the development of eurythmy from 1914 to 1919, are the photos.

On one side of the room a little staircase led up to an alcove, and through an opening in the back wall one could see part of the inside of the large cupola. From up there, one had a grand overview of a whole world speaking through a wealth of colours and forms – 'a perfectly formed world of beauty,' as Marie Steiner so aptly said. For those few still alive on earth who experienced the eurythmy room and the first Goetheanum, the memory remains vivid.

Cupboards had been built in the walls to the left and the right, and in these were kept the costumes from Steiner's Mystery Dramas and the Munich dramas of Eduard Schuré. Steiner also set aside a small room for me just off the main space. It was somewhere I could keep all the books and notebooks I needed for the lessons, and where I could sit between rehearsals and lessons to rest or prepare for the next lesson.

But all of this was lost to the fire on that tragic New Year's Eve in 1922. Nothing could be saved from the burning room. Some of our eurythmy costumes, a few dresses and veils that were kept next to the stage, were saved thanks to the courage and presence of mind of members who managed to snatch them from the flames at the last minute. Steiner later wrote about that night:

> On December 31, smoke from the fire, which grew and eventually destroyed the entire Goetheanum, was first discovered in this room. One can feel, if one was lovingly connected to this building, the merciless flames painfully penetrating the feelings that had been poured into the room's resting forms and then into the work that had been done there.[7]

The first performances

We now began the energetic working through of an immense amount of material, staging the results of our work for local and visiting anthroposophists in our weekly performances. Marie Steiner put together the programs and, with a few exceptions, recited texts for the performances. One such exception was a performance of Schiller's poem 'Ode to Joy' (done with red curtains and red lighting!), which was recited by Max Schuurman and Jan Stuten. According to Rudolf Steiner it should be done loudly, with the two of them at times almost shouting, not in the sense of naturalistic shouting, but rather as an intensification of dramatic enunciation within the limits of speech formation. We eurythmists moved correspondingly. For example, in the short pauses of *EVOE*, we made the *V* behind the head, not facing forward but with our backs to the audience. Our musicians, Leopold van der Pals, Max Schuurman, and Jan Stuten, composed musical accompaniments at this time for all the geometric forms, from triangle and square up to the eight-sided figure, as well as for all the Preludes that we had worked on in the August/September course.

Somewhat later, a form for the Humorous Introduction was added. Jan Stuten composed the music, a truly inspired piece that fully suited the style of a humoresque. For many years, the humorous part at the end of the eurythmy program always began with this Introduction. Rudolf Steiner was insistent that, even during the war, no program should omit the humorous part.

Form for the 'Humorous Introduction'
The original drawing for this form was lost in the fire that destroyed the first Goetheanum. The reproduction included here is from my own drawing; all eurythmy schools own a photocopy of it. The smaller forms that make up this Introduction are all done at the same time, with the performers repeating them many times backwards and forwards.

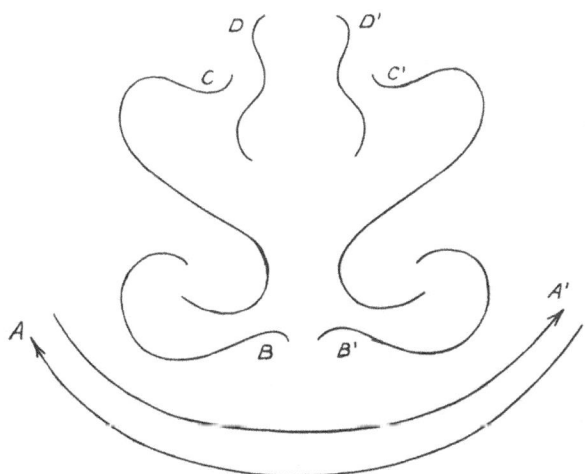

After the opening of the First Goetheanum on September 26, 1920, in accordance with Rudolf Steiner's wishes, there was a long intermission following the first part of the eurythmy performance. The audience then moved from the building over to the Carpenter's Shop where Marie Steiner introduced the final humoresque part, which always with the Introduction in tone eurythmy (only the 'Song of Initiation' was ever performed in the Goetheanum itself). It was a Polish artist with a great talent for the humorous who started the era of humoresques in eurythmy, and since then they have played an important role in performances in Dornach.

Rudolf Steiner indicated that the humorous element makes the soul life healthy and frees the human being from sentimentality. Humoresques therefore need a lot of spirit! A fine humour that avoided exaggeration thus came into its own in eurythmy, infused with a certain zest that Steiner himself supplied on a number of occasions. It should be noted that this is something different from the grotesque, which sadly attracts eurythmists as well as a larger part of audiences. How easy it is to cross over from the humorous into the grotesque. As I have done many humoresques by Christian Morgenstern, I am well aware of the danger.

The microcosmic dance
A semi-circular podium was built with three steps for the presentation of poems and of Steiner's microcosmic dance, which reproduces the organisation of the human head and larynx.

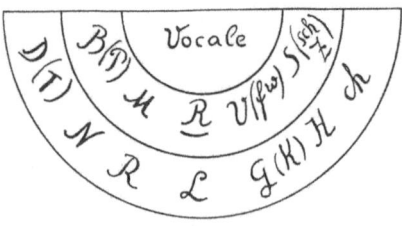

One or more eurythmists stand on the top step of the podium performing vowels and radial forms in space. In terms of Apollonian forms, that means verbs and concrete nouns. On the middle step, the consonants are performed: *B* (*P*), *M*, *R* (*R* that leans towards *A*), *V* (*F*, *W*), *S*, (*SH*, *Z*), and in standing the adjectives, conjunctions, and prepositions. On the third step, the lowest step, the consonants *D* (*T*), *N*, *R* (a short, resounding *R*), *L*, *G* (*K*), *H*, *CH* (as in *Ich*) are performed, and all forms that are curved. These are done in connection with words whose content points towards the abstract, the spiritual or the soul. This represents what is closest to the human organism: the faculty of speech. In this representation one is closest to the microcosm, just as one is closest to the macrocosm in the dance of the planets. This is how the whole human larynx is organised.

In a lecture he gave in Dornach on December 18, 1921, Steiner described the connections between the human being and the World-All or cosmos. In earlier times, the human being revealed the secret of their soul and spirit through their speech. The mystery of the human being, their relationship to the cosmos and their rootedness in the World-All, could be brought to expression in a way that was similar to what was revealed in the heavens through the fixed stars and the moving planets. This original, archetypal faculty of expression, this human word of truth or wisdom-word, has been lost. Through occult schooling, however, the human being can perceive what lies beneath the threshold of ordinary consciousness. They can experience in their etheric and physical bodies a resounding of the music of the spheres which they experienced in the spiritual world before their present earthly life. According to Steiner, the human being carries unconsciously in their physical body a reflection of the cosmic *world-consonance* as a result of the pre-earthly influence of the zodiac, and in their etheric body they carry a reflection of the cosmic *world-vocalism* (what is vowel-like) through the influence of the planets. Steiner went on to say:

> This remains, one might say, in the silence of the subconscious. But as the child develops, forces press upwards within the body and strengthen the speech organs; these are forces that, as *reflections*

of the formative forces of the cosmos, built up the speech organs. The more interior speech organs are so formed out of the human being's essential being that they can produce vowels, and the organs nearer to the periphery, the palate, the tongue, the lips and everything that contributes to the form of the physical body, are built up in such a way that consonants can be produced. While the child is learning to speak, something takes place in the upper part of their being, as a result of the activity of his lower part, which is a consequence of the formative forces taken up into the physical body. (This is naturally not a material process but has to do with formative activity.) Thus when we speak, we bring to manifestation what we might call an echo of the experience we undergo in the life between death and a new birth during our descent out of the divine spiritual world... The human being is a microcosm picture of the reality of the macrocosm.[8]

More scenes from Faust, *1916–18*

The performances of *Faust* took place at the same time as the Apollonian course in eurythmy. To this day I still feel joy and a great warmth whenever I think back on the first performances of those scenes. We had only a few days to prepare them, and at first I did not know how we could achieve this. For some reason Rudolf and Marie Steiner decided to take a step back so that we would have to do this without their help. Even the costumes (to be used for the first time in our work on *Faust*) had to be devised by us. The only suggestion Steiner made was for the 'Romantic Walpurgis Night', from *Faust: Part One*, which we performed in December 1916. He said that the ladies who were to perform the witches should all dress very individually, but not so the warlocks. The warlocks, he explained, were not human souls on the astral plane, as is the case with the witches, but rather the unconscious projections of the witches' desires. This was how they would like to see their life's partner: stripped of all individuality but gifted with all the qualities of a cat. Therefore the warlocks should be dressed as cats and be indistinguishable from one another.

After a lot of hard work in such a short time, we showed what we had made of this scene and the witches' costumes to Rudolf and Marie Steiner. The ladies all displayed an extraordinary gift for invention. For my part I appeared in a short blue skirt, an old cardigan with big holes at the elbows, and a colourfully embroidered apron. I wore a pair of broad slippers that were almost falling off my feet, and my hair was long and unkempt. I carried a big broom in my hand. The others were dressed even more fantastically! Against all expectations everything went smoothly, and we performed the whole scene with great verve. Before the entrance of Mephistopheles and Faust we danced a series of dances with the warlocks accompanied by music: solos, duets and trios, which led into a big in- and out-winding spiral movement.

Rudolf Steiner was amused by all of this. Marie Steiner also approved on the whole, although she thought that it was a little too wild. In an attempt to soften the effect, she suggested that I change my costume. The next day, before the dress rehearsal, I received a parcel from Fraülein Lehman with my new clothes: a somewhat longer skirt, a white apron, and a few other items. But whatever I tried on did not feel convincing. Marie Steiner just laughed and called out, 'Kisseleff, wear your old rags; it was much better yesterday.'

How sorry I am that no one took any photographs of us. What a colourful, fantastic company we were!

I describe this in detail because when the scene was rehearsed again in 1936, a few of the eurythmists in Dornach were of the opinion that my direction was lacking. They thought the witches should complement the warlocks, which would mean that together they would portray a sort of group soul.

They wanted every witch to look like each other, without individuality, and to be as grotesque as the witch in the 'Witch's Kitchen' scene. But Steiner wanted contrasts as well as parallels, and he cut out the part where one witch rides on a pig because he considered it too grotesque for the stage.

I believe we are obligated to preserve the characteristic directions that Steiner gave us, especially in cases such as this where the unconscious impulses of the human soul are made visible through them. I hope this example serves as a warning not to rely solely on intellectually constructed ideas when solving artistic problems. It is better to wait until the time comes that one has matured to spiritual insight.

The performance itself was again very lively and done with equal verve. A group of friends volunteered to make all sorts of noises offstage with the help of sheet metal and other objects. A few knowledgeable ones imitated a frog concert, and Steiner told them to increase the volume when Faust says, 'Songs are these? In murmurs dreaming? / Airs are these of lovers' yearning'. Faust and Mephistopheles had to move in zigzag forms as they followed the will-o'-the-wisps, and accompany the words they spoke with eurythmy gestures: Faust with vowels, Mephistopheles with consonants. With the further development of the art of speech formation, it became possible to do justice to the spiritual character of this scene through a more perfected style of speech, without needing the accompanying eurythmy gestures.

In connection with this scene Steiner said that every year, during the night of April 30 to May 1, this Walpurgis Night could be experienced on the astral plane. Souls can be seen streaming from all sides, their costumes and behaviour revealing what is living, mostly unconscious, in their natures: one can see, for example, many proud, shining queens with crowns and costly jewels, followed by a crowd of pages and admirers.

In 1917 we performed the 'Cathedral' scene, also from *Faust: Part One*. Marie Steiner recited the text, while the performer playing Gretchen did eurythmy. The part of the Evil Spirit was also done in eurythmy with vowels for the sung text and consonants for the spoken text. The performer stood on a raised pedestal and wore a broad, winged costume that had been made according to Steiner's indications.

In December 1918, the 'Classical Walpurgis Night' scene from *Faust: Part Two* was performed. This was a major event in the development of eurythmy in relation to drama. The preparation lasted many months. Marie Steiner worked with us on the group dances, especially the one for the Lamiae, the child-devouring female demons. Many interesting ideas came to her for the forms; when we moved around the figures of Empuse and Mephistopheles, she divided us into ever-changing groups that resulted in unexpected combinations.

Behind the scenes, in the costume studio, there appeared in quick succession sphinxes, griffins, ants, the Phorkyaden, dolphins, and all the various wonders of the sea that have enchanted audiences at the Goetheanum ever since. The appearance of each individual creature backstage was a joyful experience for all who participated in the stage work and was the pride of their creators: Bertha Ellram, who was in charge of the wardrobe at that time, and her helpers. Rudolf Steiner gave indications for the costumes and continuously checked the results.

During the rehearsals, Steiner spoke about the characters of the various beings, and Marie Steiner worked tirelessly with trained helpers to express their individualities through spoken recitation. Leopold van der Pals composed the music for the sirens and other parts. In the Carpenter's Shop and neighbouring rooms every corner was occupied by single groups practising. Here the sirens were learning their tones; there the Tritons were holding their tridents; in another corner the fisher boys were quickly learning their vowels; farther off were the Nereids and Dorids, and children practising the ants, pygmies and daktyls. Away from the rest, in the eurythmy room in the Goetheanum, the performers of the Phorkyads sat for hours, practising their special gestures.

Once all of these various elements were completed (including, in the end, the carriage with the shell for Galatea), the whole sequence of the 'Classical Walpurgis Night' was staged in the Carpenter's Shop, which had been enlarged for this purpose. At first it was performed only for members and but then later also for the general public.

During this period Rudolf Steiner gave many lectures on Goethe's *Faust* that cast light on the scenes being performed from an anthroposophical point of view.[9] On January 16, 1919, the 'Classical Walpurgis Night' scene was performed for those interned in the First World War. In his introductory words, Steiner pointed out that these scenes bring to expression Goethe's spiritual life in his most mature years, and that for Goethe, the riddle of knowledge flows together with the artistic element in a most inspired way. After another performance on Christmas Day, he said that eurythmy is particularly well-suited to presenting this powerful Goethean creation of art and knowledge.

The eurythmy dress

In the autumn of 1918, before leaving Dornach for a few weeks, Steiner asked us to think about what the right garment for eurythmy should be. On his return, we gathered on the stage in the Carpenter's Shop to show him our results. Of the ten dresses on show, he pointed to one and said, 'That is the eurythmy dress!' It was the dress that I happened to be wearing and I would like to relate quite candidly how I came to it.

Until shortly before Steiner's return, I still had not come up with a design for the right eurythmy dress. Then an idea came to me suddenly: I saw a beautiful white garment floating down towards me, as though descending from heavenly heights. Filled with joy I set to work to make my vision a reality. This would be the standard dress for our Dornach eurythmy group for many years. It was cut out of a light silk material, long and wide, and had many folds, both in the top and in the skirt. It was sewn in one piece. It had an elastic band drawn through the hem at the neck and waist, as well as long, wide sleeves. A large, thin veil was worn over the dress. A long skirt made out of a thick material was worn as an undergarment to conceal the shape of the eurythmist's legs as much as possible. Rudolf Steiner was very strict on this point. The stockings and light eurythmy shoes (without heels) were the same colour as the dress. Only on a few occasions were the stockings a different colour, and then mainly in humoresques. On no account were we allowed to do eurythmy barefoot. On the other hand, the veils were often a different colour from the dress. On tours, every eurythmist took a number of wide skirt-like trousers of various colours that ended a little below the knee. These were used as undergarments for the coloured dresses that were added over time to the white ones. In those days, great effort was made to follow this indication, although nowadays it is scorned by many eurythmists.

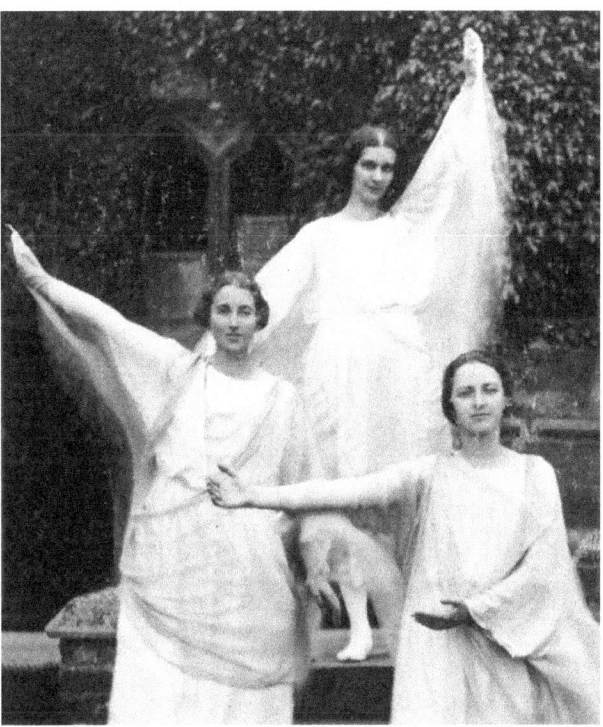

Oxford, 1923. From left to right: Flossie Leinhaus-von Sonclar, Tatiana Kisseleff, and Ilse Kimball-von Baravalle. They are wearing the dress designed by Tatiana Kisseleff.

1918–19: Stepping Out in Public

At the end of 1918, after the previously mentioned scenes from *Faust* had been performed, I frequently thought that I had completed my task in Dornach. I told myself that there were now a sufficient number of trained eurythmists in Dornach who could give lessons, and that I should withdraw from teaching and performing and do something else. I was too one-sided in my development and felt ignorant about a great many things. I was too unworldly and lacking a deeper understanding of other human beings: their lives, their various professions, and all the hard work they did for others. I spoke to Marie Steiner about this, and she invited me to tell Rudolf Steiner about my intentions over supper. Steiner asked me what I wanted to do. I answered that I was not yet clear, but that I often had the idea of doing practical work of some sort, in a factory perhaps. But Steiner responded that my health would not allow me to do heavy physical work. And so, that evening, I decided to expand our eurythmy activity by taking it out into the world. To begin with, we would perform at the Pfauen Theatre in Zürich, but eventually our little ship would leave the calm waters of Dornach and venture, boldly and courageously, on our first pioneering journey to further parts of the world.

The Pfauen Theatre, Zürich

The first eurythmy performance in the Pfauen Theatre was scheduled for the end of 1918, but was postponed until

February 24, 1919. At Rudolf Steiner's request Walo von May, a Swiss painter who was deeply connected to eurythmy, designed a poster that was hung in the streets of Zürich and in bookstores and public buildings a few days before the performance. The colour drawing was also included in the performance program. Thanks to his strong intuitive gift, Walo von May was able to capture and express the spiritual aspect of this event. In the picture everything is in movement. The new-born child 'Eurythmy' calls forth the strongest reaction: on the one hand, there are the enthusiastic cheers of the sounding, light-filled world; on the other, there is the chaos and revolt of the frightened beings of darkness. The large pink figure holds the child 'Eurythmy' to her heart. Below the child is a human figure who forms the sounds of the introductory *TIAOAIT* in eurythmy, which was to be the first thing the audience saw at the performance in Zürich.

I have seldom seen Steiner so radiant as on the day he appeared in the Carpenter's Shop holding the poster in his hand. He showed it to us and expressed his satisfaction at such a successful work of art.

Before the performance in the Pfauen Theatre Steiner spoke briefly about the basic intentions of eurythmy as an art form. Marie Steiner recited all the poems. The large audience who attended this first performance did so with interest and, for the most part, with good will.

The first items on the program were received in a mood of expectation and complete silence, which was probably due more to surprise than anything else. The first item on the program was 'Words to the Spirit and to Love' from scene 3 of *The Portal of Initiation* ('Light's weaving essence...'), with the form *TIAOAIT* and music by Leopold van der Pals. The title, 'Words to the Spirit and to Love', was first given by Rudolf Steiner to this verse for this performance. We performed the text with Apollonian forms and the appropriate vowels, moving with great animation to the next part of the form only during the pauses in which Marie Steiner took a breath. Rudolf Steiner

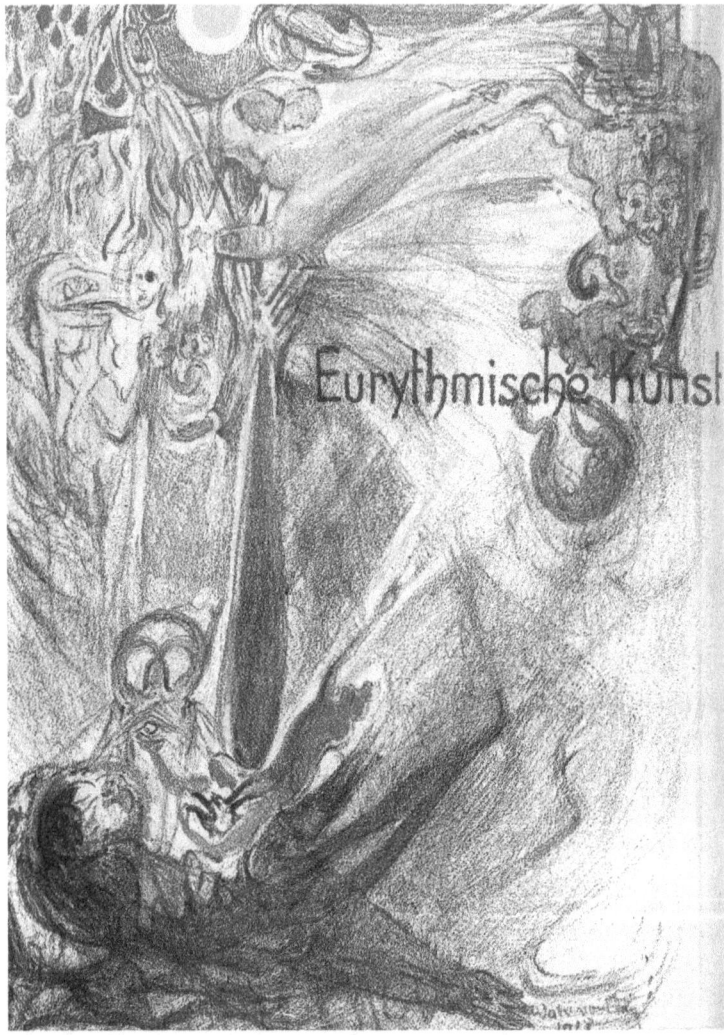

The drawing by Walo von May for the first public eurythmy performance in Zürich in 1919.

wanted the transitions to be 'quick and lively but without haste'. The third item on the program was the 'Dance of the Planets', beginning with the line 'The Sun is shining.' After these first pieces, the audience applauded enthusiastically, acknowledging our young art that was so different from anything they had seen in the realm of dance until that moment.

It was with this beginning that eurythmy was placed before

the audience in its true, deeper nature as the new art of the Mysteries.

Marie Steiner writes the following in the introduction to the book *Eurythmy as Visible Speech*:

> After many years of ceaseless training and appearances in performances with like-minded people, the performers of eurythmy were able to present their work to the public. The reactions were strong: they found either enthusiastic responses or passionate antagonism. No one remained indifferent. The cultural dictators threatened ostracism; the press were usually told to write against it, even when, as many admitted, they felt personally enthusiastic about it. Those representing the neighbouring arts were often deeply moved, but also often aggressively ironical. Those from the stream of reformers felt their thought-out systems threatened by an unknown, but certainly forward-looking power. Unprejudiced audiences thanked God that there could be such a pure and noble art. Children usually asked whether they were the angels they had heard about and those carried away by enthusiasm uttered loud '*ahs*' and '*ohs*' as an indication of the impression it made on them. This art worked within the swamp of our modern civilization like a light and as a flame; in between, some dark night birds shrieked and reviled as if they were being purified in a bath of steel. Others who wanted to escape the decline of our culture felt able to breathe. The spirit forged a path into an art which worked to both cleanse and animate.[1]

That first performance in Zürich was the biggest, most joyful day of my life, my day of destiny. I was filled with deepest gratitude, and felt certain that many in the audience had been yearning for a long time for a more spiritual form of dance. It seemed to me that many left the performance relieved and full of joy, carrying hope in their souls.

Naturally, there were many who were unhappy that the anthroposophists who, until now, had kept quietly out of the way in Dornach, had suddenly took it upon themselves to appear in public. The press, as was expected of them, reacted more or less disapprovingly, although it is interesting to compare two comments that appeared in two different newspapers on the presentation of the *Hallelujah* that followed the poem 'On the Sistine Madonna' by Hebbel. The critic of one newspaper described it as a badly done gymnastic exercise, whereas the critic in the other wrote that he was deeply moved by it and felt his soul lifted up out of everyday profane life into Manichean spiritual heights!

This performance inaugurated a new period of eurythmy activity. It continued with public performances in the Carpenter's Shop and the Goetheanum itself, followed by a series of pioneering tours in towns around Germany, Austria, Czechoslovakia, Norway, England, Holland, and Switzerland.

Introduction from the Pfauen Theatre programme:

The art of movement known as eurythmy, which until now has only been cultivated in intimate circles, has its origin in the Goethean view that all art is the revelation of natural laws that would remain hidden but for art's revelation. Another thought from Goethe can be connected with this one, namely, that in every individual organ in the human being, one can find a lawful expression of the whole human being. Every single member of the human being is to some extent a human being in miniature, just as, Goetheanistically speaking, the leaf of a plant is the whole plant in miniature. One can also reverse this thought and thereby see in the whole human being a complete expression of what each one of their organs represents. Speaking, singing and movement (or the tendency toward movement) are

Montag, den 24. Februar 1919, abends 8 Uhr, findet im
PFAUENTHEATER eine Darstellung

EURYTHMISCHER KUNST

statt. Sie wird veranstaltet sein durch

TATIANA KISSELEFF

unter Mitwirkung von Elisabeth Dollfuß, Anna Marie Groh,
Anna Marie Donath, Edith Röhrle u. a.

Die der Aufführung zu Grunde liegenden
Dichtungen werden von Marie Steiner re=
zitiert, die begleitende Musik ist von Leopold
van der Pals, von Max Schuurman, Jan Stuten

Die eurythmische Kunstform ist nach Intentionen und Angaben Rudolf Steiners gebildet

Karten zu 3.—, 4.—, 5.— und 6.— Fr. Billetverkauf an der Theaterkasse abends 7 Uhr. Vorverkauf am 22., 23. und 24. Februar 1919
von 11½—12½ Uhr an der Theaterkasse

Der Feurich=Konzertflügel stammt aus dem Pianohaus Jecklin, Zürich

PROGRAMM

Einleitende Worte v. Rudolf Steiner über eurytmische Kunst

In eurythmischer Einzel- oder Gruppenkunst kommen zur Darstellung:

Worte an den Geist und die Liebe.. aus Rudolf Steiners „Pforte der Einweihung", mit musikalischer Beigabe von L. van der Pals . . . . dargestellt durch eine Gruppe

Was treibt du, Wind .. v. Konrad Ferd. Meyer . E. Dollfuss u. A. Groh

Planetentanz .. v. Rudolf Steiner, mit musik. Auftakt v. L. van der Pals . . . . eine Gruppe

Göttermahl .. v. K. Ferd. Meyer, mit musik. Beigabe von L. v. der Pals . . . . eine Gruppe

Noch einmal.. von Konrad Ferdinand Meyer, mit musikalischem Auftakt von L. van der Pals . . . . Tatiana Kisseleff

Auftakt „Schau um dich, schau in dich" v. L. van der Pals . eine Gruppe

Vor den Pforten des Paradieses .. v. Hans Reinhart . eine Gruppe

Auf die Sixtinische Madonna .. v. Friedr. Hebbel . Tatiana Kisseleff

Halleluja .. Eurythmie ohne Worte . . . . eine Gruppe

Aus dem „Chor der Urtriebe" .. v. Ferd. v. Steinwand . eine Gruppe

Der Musensohn .. von Wolfgang Goethe mit musikalischem Auftakt von L. van der Pals . . . . eine Gruppe

PAUSE

Vereinsamt .. von Friedrich Nietsche, mit musikalischer Beigabe von L. van der Pals . . . . eine Gruppe

Jahreszeiten .. von Hans Reinhart . . . . eine Gruppe

Elfenmusik .. von Jan Stuten . . . .

Liederseelen .. von Konrad Ferdinand Meyer . . . . eine Gruppe

Haidenröslein .. von Wolfgang Goethe, mit musikalischem Auftakt von Jan Stuten . . . . Tatiana Kisseleff und Elisabeth Dollfuss

Die gebratene Flunder .. von Paul Scheerbart, mit musikalischem Auftakt von L. van der Pals . . . . eine Gruppe

Km 21 . . . .
Bim bam bum . . . . } aus Christians Morgensterns „Galgenliedern" . . . . eine Gruppe
Das aesthetische Wiesel

Der Tanz .. v. Friedrich Schiller, mit musikalischer Beigabe von Max Schuurman . . . . eine Gruppe

carried out in the larynx and the organs connected with it, and these are revealed in sounds and the connections of sounds that go unobserved in everyday life. Not so much the movements themselves, but rather the intention behind the movement is now transposed in eurythmy into movements of the whole body. What takes place imperceptibly when forming speech sounds and musical tones with the speech organs, becomes visible through the movement and bearing of the whole human being. Movements of the human limbs reveal what takes place in the larynx and neighbouring organs in speaking and singing. Movement through space and in group forms and movements express what is living in the human soul in music and speech. Thereby the impulses which have worked in the creation of all forms of art have prevailed in the creation of this eurythmical art of movement. Arbitrary miming or pantomime or symbolic soul expression in movement is not included. Expressiveness is achieved through lawful inner relationships, as in music. Eurythmy leads back to what the art of dance once took as its point of departure in the nature of the artistic, and from which it has moved away in the course of time. It wants to do this in the sense of a truly modern conception of art, not through an imitation or mere reconstruction of the past. It lies in the nature of the thing that the art of eurythmy connects itself to the musical. Musical pieces that appear in the course of the eurythmy program were composed by Leopold van der Pals, Max Schuurman, and Jan Stuten. What now appears as eurythmy is a beginning; the intentions connected to this art will eventually find their further development. However, they would like to be taken up as a beginning.*

Further work in the Carpenter's Shop

Before going on to describe the period of our eurythmy tours, I would like to mention a few other things that happened around this time.

There were many members in Dornach who, for various

reasons, had been unable to participate in the eurythmy courses. A communal course was therefore offered for this large group of friends, made up of the old, the young, and all ages in between. The course took place in the Carpenter's Shop, where many enjoyable social events took place. The lessons were well attended and we often had forty, fifty, or even sixty people at a time. Mothers brought their small children with them, unable to leave them at home, and while the mothers joined in the exercises, the children were often passed from one person to another.

There was a eurythmy group for children as well. We worked on fairy tales and performed them on the stage in the Carpenter's Shop for the parents and their friends. For the little children these were often more than just plays. When we did 'Snow White and the Seven Dwarves', they wept real tears when Snow White bit into the poisoned apple and fell down as though dead, and let out great cries of joy when she was awoken by the prince. A low table was then placed on the stage and the children sat themselves around it on small benches to celebrate the wedding of the hero of the fairy tale. They were served hot chocolate and cakes, which had been prepared off stage in a little room adjoining the stage. One could hear them chatting and dividing up the roles amongst themselves: 'I want to be the cobbler for the princess,' 'I want to be the prince's cook!' and so on. Then a chain was formed and the hero of the fairy tale led the procession around the building, ending at the canteen at the foot of the hill. A lady had put Snow White into verse, so the presentation was accompanied by recitation and music and performed in eurythmy by the children.

Another project took place in the Carpenter's Shop in the summer of 1918. Rudolf and Marie Steiner were absent from Dornach for a few months. Because there were no lectures happening at this time, some of the members who had not had much of a chance to learn about eurythmy, expressed the wish to familiarise themselves with the content of the 1915 course, both theoretically and practically. This was done through a series of presentations, beginning each time with a talk about

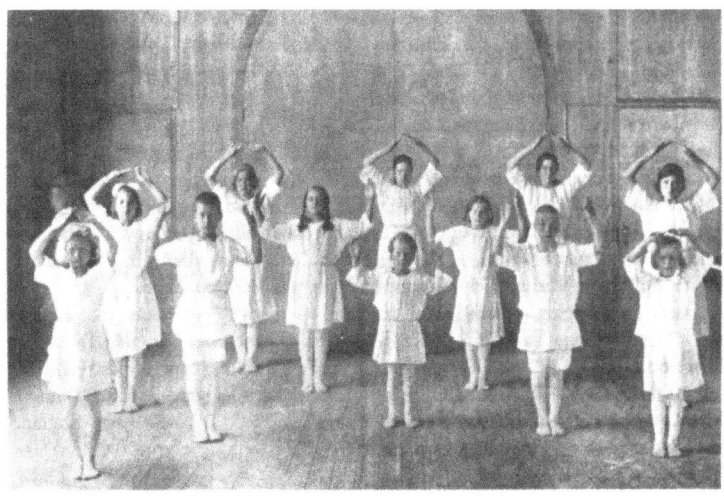

Children performing eurythmy in the Carpenter's Shop in Dornach.

the essence of Apollonian eurythmy, followed immediately by a form drawn on the blackboard to make it visible. An appropriate poem was then performed on the stage in the Carpenter's Shop.

For several weeks during June and July we worked on the problem of expressing colours in eurythmy. In the 1915 course Steiner had indicated how the human hand, in its relationship to the arm, could express the spectrum of colours. When dealing with this or that colour, there would usually be a demonstration of a number of colour poems before the theory was presented. Chapters from Goethe's *Theory of Colours*, especially the chapter on the moral associations of colours, were discussed, as well as Steiner's expansion and deepening of Goethe's original ideas: for example, in the lecture he gave on January 1, 1915, 'Moral Experience of the Worlds of Colour and Tone'.[2] We also discussed his lectures on the Bhagavad-Gita in which he describes humanity's path from light into darkness at the time of the Mystery of Golgotha.[3] The culmination of this work was a performance of a few rainbow poems.

When Rudolf and Marie Steiner returned we showed them the results of our work. Among the many poems we had worked on was Schiller's poem 'The Riddle', and the verse that begins, 'We children six our being had / From a most strange and wondrous pair.' Rudolf Steiner changed the first line to, 'We seven, we are world sisters...'

The fundamental idea of Goethe's colour theory, that colours come into existence through the interaction of light and dark, was indicated by the two figures that Steiner added to the other seven. The mother stood downstage on the left, dressed completely in black, and the father downstage on the right dressed completely in white. The mother did the dark vowels and the father the light sounds in the lines that had to do with them. In the middle, between the two, the agile dance of the seven sisters took place, each with their individual colours. The beginning position of the nine figures as given by Steiner, along with their corresponding colours and vowels, was as follows:

Mother = black   A = blue   E = orange

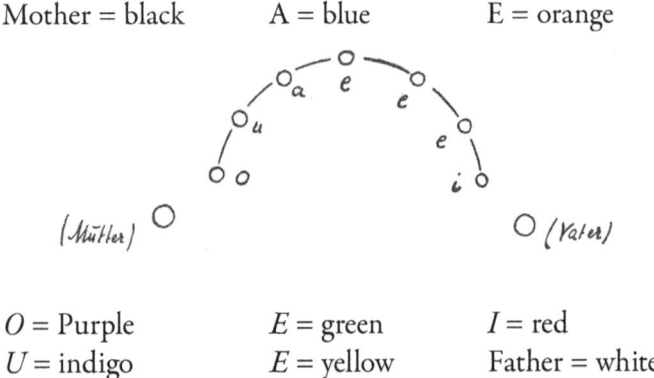

O = Purple   E = green   I = red
U = indigo   E = yellow   Father = white

We also did a performance of Goethe's poem 'Rain and Rainbow'. Mieta Pyle-Waller played the philistine, who grumbles and philosophises about the uselessness of the rainbow. During the dress rehearsal, Steiner asked her to wear his coat, hat and boots and, with his umbrella, to do eurythmy as she walked around at the back of the stage. The effect of her appearance in the performance the next day was sensational. The other seven ladies, representing the rainbow, were each draped with a veil in one of the seven colours.

During the early development of eurythmy, the staging of dramatic scenes often underwent dramatic changes themselves. For example, at the beginning of 'The Dying Medusa', by Conrad Ferdinand Meyer, the Medusa had to lie outstretched on the stage. Above her, standing on an elevation indicating a rock, was Perseus dressed in a Greek tunic and performing eurythmy with a sword in his right hand. During the course of the poem the Medusa got up, acted her role at the front of the stage and then approached Perseus, sinking down slowly as she died. All of this was done in eurythmy. Later on, however, Rudolf Steiner gave new forms for both figures. The eurythmists were also given purely eurythmical costumes, and the naturalistic sword and stage directions were abolished.

The same was done with other poems too. The props that were used in Goethe's poem 'Charon', such as cymbals and the hammer, disappeared in order to make way for eurythmy in its truest form. Naturalistic action was dispensed with and expressed in other ways. For example, bending the knees was intended to represent memory or an expression of the past, while going up on the tips of one's toes was a gesture of situating oneself in the future. Bending or performing a graceful jump was used for exclamations and feelings. Other gestures and actions were likewise derived from the same non-naturalistic principle.

Through the art of eurythmy, through the different movements of the limbs and the corresponding forms in space, quite other possibilities are available for expressing the soul-spiritual element than existed before. In earlier times human beings could only achieve this by using objects. According to Steiner, in the ancient temple dances participants carried branches, the buds expressing the mood of Mars (see p. 174, The World Clock, on the connection of Mars to the sound I). Although eurythmy is not a repetition of those earlier temple dances, Steiner said that moving with a rod created a lightening effect in the surrounding aura, and the rod could be replaced by a branch, either budding or evergreen. However, in the new dance of the planets that he gave us, Steiner recommended that we not use any objects. Indeed, we never used flowers of any kind in Dornach even when flowers were mentioned in a poem, except in the Burial Scene in *Faust: Part Two* when angels scatter roses to prevent Mephistopheles and the devils from seizing Faust's soul. Instead, through a deep experience of the sounds – for example, through the correct unfolding of the *L* – we endeavoured to come close to the being of the flower itself, echoing what Steiner meant when he said:

> When we enter into the tulip blossom with our soul forces we express, in the Imagination of the tulip, what is expressed here on the Earth in the formation of words. We grow again into the spiritual aspect of everything.[4]

At the beginning of his instruction in eurythmy, Steiner did indicate a group of consonants that were to be done 'with a foreign object'. These were *V, B, S* and *T*. In a poem with this group of consonants one could use a veil, which must hang loosely over the dress, or another object. This would in no way go against what is understood as pure eurythmy. These are the fine distinctions that need to be made.

Eurythmy had to go through this transitional stage. As Steiner said in his introductory words to the eurythmy performance given on July 1, 1923:

> The development of eurythmy happened in this way, that its true character emerged over the course of years. In this way an art of movement came into being that could only arise out of the anthroposophical movement as conceived of for the new age, for the present and near future.[5]

The visit of some forty children from Vienna to Dornach in 1921 was a delight for all of us. They stayed with anthroposophists and others living nearby, and I gave them eurythmy lessons every day. The children grew to love the work. They made such a great effort that at the end of six weeks, before their return to Vienna, we could put on a performance on the stage in the Carpenter's Shop.

From the start Rudolf Steiner followed our work with children with great interest. Already in the winter of 1915, while the eurythmy room was still being built, he had offered the dining room and entrance hall of this house, Villa Hansi, for eurythmy lessons. We could come any time, he told us, but we would need to give him and Marie a day's notice so that they could move the furniture and prepare the space. When I expressed my concern that the noise of the children would disturb him, he answered with his radiant smile, 'No, on the contrary.'

Steiner would sometimes come down near the end of the children's lessons to watch them perform. He would joke with them and engage them in conversation. On one occasion he said to a five-year-old boy who did nothing but disturb the others, 'You are not in the picture!' When I asked him what I should do to stop the boy from being so disruptive, Steiner said that although he appeared to be doing nothing, the boy was in fact watching my movements and learning from them. No doubt he would decide to join in soon enough. And it proved to be true. The next lesson the boy placed himself obediently 'in the picture'. He did threefold walking and the golden mean gestures for the rhythms and vowels perfectly – much to the amazement of the other children. After that he took part in lessons with all his heart and soul.

The Dornach children's group also visited various Swiss towns to give performances, and in his introductions Steiner often spoke about the pedagogical and artistic elements of eurythmy. In a lecture he gave in Dornach he said that when children perform eurythmy they enable divine spiritual beings to work into them, and that this helps the children grow into life in the right way.

Sometimes Steiner would appear in the Carpenter's Shop carrying some small child in his arms whom he had 'abducted'

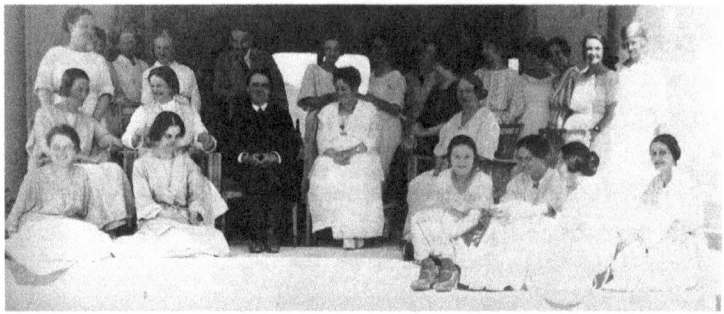

Rudolf and Marie Steiner surrounded by the eurythmy group outside Haus Duldeck in Dornach in 1921. Tatiana Kisseleff is in the front row, second from the left.

from their mother. The child would observe everything that was happening around them, full of trust, with Steiner's loving gaze resting on them.

The experience of working in the Carpenter's Shop was truly unique. Rehearsals took place in an atmosphere of soul-spiritual inwardness and with a wonderful childlike solemnity. The majority of eurythmists whom destiny had brought together were at that time between twenty and thirty years old, some were not even twenty and only the very oldest were a little over thirty. So it was a rather young group of artists. But this was not the reason for the unique atmosphere. This must be attributed to the special natures of Rudolf and Marie Steiner who guided the work and in whom there worked and weaved the same forces they sought to awaken in us through eurythmy.

As Steiner had said in a previous lecture, eurythmy is a means of awakening the forces that we retain from earliest childhood when we learn to walk, forces that go unnoticed later on in life. Eurythmy can help us train these forces and use them to see into the spiritual realm in which we live between death and rebirth. These forces are the most innocent forces that we possess. They play into the aura of a child and are full of wisdom; they are what makes the appearance of a child so enchanting to us. This is what lies behind the words in Matthew's Gospel, 'Unless you change and become like little children, you will never enter the kingdom of heaven.'[6]

Rudolf Steiner speaks about the mystery of getting younger

as one grows older in the lectures about the youth forces in human nature. The mystery of rejuvenation lies in the wisdom of the head becoming deepened through the life of the heart, transformed through the love rising up out of the whole human being. This rejuvenating transformation can come about in a person who has understood how to maintain inner liveliness and mobility of soul throughout their life:

> This is exactly the task of the future, that head knowledge eventually becomes transformed through heart knowledge ... The heart will look up toward the head and will see imprinted in it the image of the starry heavens. But the head will look towards the heart and will find there the secrets of the riddles of humanity, it will come to know the essence of the human being in the heart.[7]

The strength to fulfil this future task is to be found in Benedictus's words in scene 3 of *The Portal of Initiation* where he directs Johannes Thomasius toward the spirit realm. These words formed the first item in the first eurythmy performance in Zürich, 'Words to the Spirit and to Love':

> Light's weaving essence radiates
> through far-flung spaces
> to fill the world with life.
> Love's blessing pours its warmth
> through time's long ages
> to call forth revelation of all worlds.
> And messengers of spirit join
> light's weaving essence
> with revelation of the soul.
> And when with both the human being
> can join their own true self
> they are alive in spirit heights.[8]

The secret of that magical, wonder-working atmosphere in which the eurythmy work took place in those years is therefore to be found in the presence that touched us through the agency of these two individuals, Rudolf and Marie Steiner, these bearers of spirit substance who dwelt among us as representatives of this light-filled future.

Rudolf Steiner always brought new forms for poems or musical compositions, spoke about the character of the movement in different poems, and gave lively suggestions for humoresques. His forms, composed in a variety of individual and increasingly differentiated ways, grew to form a wonderful, harmonious whole in which each one was itself a complete and perfect work of art. It made you want to gaze upon these countless pages again and again with their beautifully drawn lines that came from the hand of the master.

A unique moral and social impulse streamed out from this work. It is difficult to speak about it because of the many imponderables that played invisibly and inaudibly between the souls of the people who took part in it. Rudolf and Marie Steiner not only encouraged artistic abilities, but in the broadest and deepest sense they influenced the growth of a true humanity in each one of us. Steiner often walked through the different areas backstage and spoke to the workers who were diligently sewing, mending, dusting and washing the floors, people who were not usually seen by the audience. He thanked them and encouraged them in their labours.

In the lectures he gave on the theme of vocation in 1916, Steiner spoke about the importance of material work and the special spirituality it contains. Although we may not be conscious of it at the present time, nevertheless such work is helping to prepare for a far-distant future of Earth evolution.[9] This brought forth a feeling of joy in the souls of those doing the so-called 'heavy work' behind the scenes and in different areas, and their faces beamed after this lecture. I often had cause to think of those days a few years later at the École Rudolf Steiner in Paris, when I had to do this 'heavy work' until late into the night because we did not have the means to hire a cleaner.

Once, after a performance of a scene from *Faust*, Steiner thanked all of the artists and applauded what they had achieved, but he also thanked those who went unseen by the audience but without whom the performance could not take place. On another occasion I remember Steiner saying to a eurythmist who was standing backstage and looking somewhat sadly at a program fixed to the wall, 'You are not in the program today – not in a single item!' Realising the opportunity this gave her, the eurythmist was suddenly joyful and helped out for the entire performance. She was happy to assist the eurythmists with changing dresses and veils between pieces.

Steiner once said to me that it must become irrelevant whether something is done by oneself or by someone else, what matters is that it is done. Sometimes, during rehearsals in the Carpenter's Shop, Marie Steiner would come and watch attentively. Afterwards she would ask, 'Who is sitting at the back?' and some unsuspecting person would suddenly find themselves with an important part in whatever new poem we were working on. Marie Steiner encouraged us and was happy when we managed to overcome any difficulty. She could be strict, as could Rudolf Steiner himself, but we felt that behind this severity there was an immense love and a wish to help. The younger generation must not think that it was easy or comfortable. We struggled hard and worked with all our strength, sometimes to the point of despair. Nothing escaped the keen eyes of Rudolf and Marie Steiner, which was reflected in the commitment and effort that lived in each one of us whenever we presented some part of our work on the stage.

There were occasions when I could only work on my eurythmy pieces at the end of my working day, which meant after 10.00 pm when the Carpenter's Shop was locked. Because of this, Steiner gave me permission to practise until 11.00 pm or later if necessary and gave instructions to the watchman to let me in at this late hour.

Work proceeded at an unbelievably fast pace. The days were filled with eurythmy lessons, rehearsals for performances, and practising big group pieces. The eurythmists and the other artists backstage – especially the wardrobe mistresses, Bertha Ellram and then, from 1920, Louise Clason, and also Käthe Mitscher, who cared for so many aspects of the organisation – worked from morning until late at night. Steiner once told us that we should not consider the day to be properly spent unless in the evening one can hardly stand on one's legs and has hardly enough energy to get to one's bed but instead falls on the floor like a sack!

Vowels and the planets

On January 3, 1918, Rudolf Steiner gave me a piece of paper on which he had written the vowels with the corresponding planets.

Saturn:	U	Saturn:	A	Moon:	$I - Ei$
Jupiter:	O	Jupiter:	E	Sun:	$I - AU$
Mars:	I	Mars:	I		
Venus:	E	Venus:	O		
Mercury:	A	Mercury:	U		

Steiner indicated that as the planets pass through the zodiac they change their vowels. Unfortunately, as was the case with the text for the 'Dance of the Sun, Moon and Earth', which he only recited, Steiner provided no written verse to accompany this. The text he handed me that day, in which each part sounds so differently, is wonderful and entirely unique.

Around this time, Steiner held a series of lectures that later appeared under the title *Mystery Truths and Christmas Impulses: Ancient Myths and their Meaning*.[10] The fourth lecture, it seems to me, solves the problem of the connection between the speech sounds and the planets, and the relationship between the planets and the signs of the zodiac. On the basis of these lectures and the drawings provided by Steiner, I became absorbed in these relationships and their meanings.

I will return to my work on the planets and the zodiac, the day and night houses, when I discuss the World Clock later on. Even though I have not progressed much further since that time, I carry them in my consciousness and feel a strong sense of duty to strive and grapple with them. One lifetime alone is not enough to work through all of these indications. Only the first preparatory work can be done now in the hope that in future lives it will be brought to maturity. An intensive study of spiritual science over many years is what is needed to begin with to permeate ourselves with its all-encompassing wisdom. Then, when we are ready, we will be able to move in spirit with the planets on their path through the zodiac, wandering from day to day, hour to hour, feeling at one with the whole movement of planetary existence.

Consonants and the zodiac

Already in 1915 Rudolf Steiner had given the first indications for assigning the twelve consonants to the twelve signs of the zodiac. Here is a sketch, given to me by Steiner in 1917, of the consonants divided according to the fixed stars. Above Aries (*W*)* and Taurus (*A*) Steiner wrote: 'These are half-consonants, vowel-like consonants.'

He also gave me the following correspondences: *A–R*, *T–D*, *B–P*, *Z–S*, *Sch*, and *V–F*.

---

* Corresponds to *V* in English.

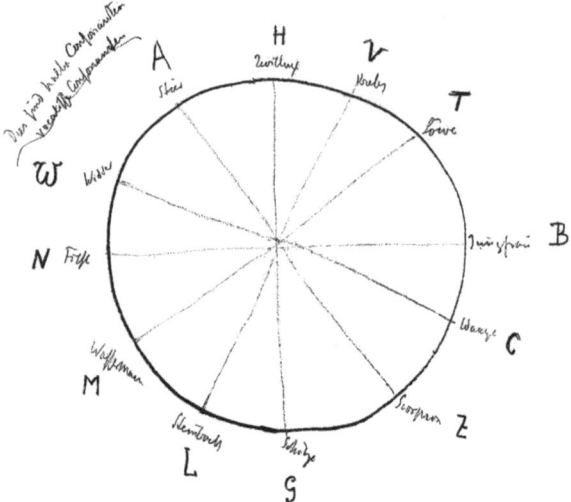

I asked how *C* (Libra) was to be done in eurythmy.

'Do it as *Z*,' Steiner replied (meaning the *ts* sound), 'but with a different starting point.'

He went on to say that because Libra was the last sign to be added to the zodiac, the consonants by then had already been divided up. For this reason one took the speech sound from the neighbouring sign Scorpio, *Z* (*ts*), for Libra as well.

I have pointed to the danger that eurythmy can degenerate into a kind of signalling, and the advice Steiner gave to counteract this. He expected all anthroposophists to work on what was given in lectures and written works until it became inner experience. The whole soul must become permeated by what is meant by spiritual science. I have tried to do this for over fifty years, especially in eurythmy and the problem of the connection between the speech sounds and the stars. Through this activity it has become clear to me that besides practising eurythmy itself, the study of the work of Rudolf Steiner, where matters are dealt with from different points of view, is imperative. This is our daily bread, our *panem supersubsantialem*.

In many lectures Steiner emphasises that human beings actually have twelve senses, we are a microcosmic picture of the macrocosm:

> In the macrocosm the sun moves through twelve
> signs of the zodiac in the course of a year, and the
> human I lives here on the physical plane in the
> twelve senses ... Our inner life moves through this
> circle of the twelve senses just as the sun moves
> through the circle of the twelve signs of the zodiac.[11]

The lecture cycle *The Spiritual Hierarchies and the Physical World* also deals with the correspondence between the human being and the twelve constellations. In the fourth lecture Steiner speaks about the original meaning of the zodiac, and in the eighth lecture we read:

> Indeed, the names of the various regions of the zodiac
> arose as a result of the human form being projected
> outward into the cosmos. It is not always easy to
> discover the original intention from the frequently
> distorted or misrepresented names [of the signs of the
> zodiac] ... In several instances, the name has not been
> handed down correctly, and so one has to go back to
> the source to obtain a clear picture.[12]
>
> For this the following paragraph is of particular
> importance.

'The Twelve Moods'

I consider it an earnest duty to take this poem, which Rudolf Steiner created and meant for performance, into one's daily eurythmy practice and to work meditatively with it. To neglect to do this would be a failing. The same laws found in the universe can also be found in the structure of this poem. Therefore, through it the human being can be connected with the great supersensible laws of the cosmos.[13]

Steiner spoke at the first performance of this poem on August 29, 1915 about the 'moving tranquillity' of the universe, the twelvefoldness of the zodiac, and the sevenfoldness of the planets and said, 'You have seen how the tranquillity of the constellations of the zodiac in comparison to the mobility of planetary existence comes out in this presentation.'

In 'The Twelve Moods' the order of the seven lines in each of the verses and their connection to a particular planetary body is as follows:

The first is the *Sun* line	AU	later	AU
The second is the *Venus* line	E	later	A
The third is the *Mercury* line	A	later	I
The fourth is the *Mars* line	I	later	E
The fifth is the *Jupiter* line	O	later	O
The sixth is the *Saturn* line	U	later	U
The seventh is the *Moon* line	EI	later	EI

The entrances and exits are as follows:

ENTRANCE   EXIT

1. Moon   7.
2. Saturn with Aries and Libra   6.
3. Jupiter with Taurus and Virgo   5.
4. Mars with Gemini and Leo   4.
5. Sun with Cancer and Capricorn   3.
6. Venus with Pisces and Scorpio   2.
7. Mercury with Aquarius and Sagittarius   1.

In the lecture he gave on July 11, 1916, Steiner says that this poem is an attempt to put into poetic form what has been drawn out of the mysteries of the World-All, what speaks in the laws of the universe:

> Thus, what is going outside in the cosmos, in the harmony of the spheres, is also in the meaning of the twelve stanzas of seven lines each. The laws of the

cosmos are meant to prevail in these twelve verses of seven lines.[14]

Working through this poem in the right way, especially with eurythmy, would lead to the ideal described by Steiner in the introduction he gave to the performance in 1915:

> Thus the ideal would actually be for someone, were they awakened from sleep and had one line read to them – 'In growing activity endures' – they would say, 'Ah, yes! Mars in Scorpio!' … What is attempted is to maintain in real, inner comprehension what was carried out cosmically when our solar system was created … it could be said that what you have seen presented here offers the possibility of creating movement, as well as concepts steeped in movement, out of what can be expressed in the following phrase: 'The word weaves through the world, and the world-formation holds the word fast.'[15]

The unjustified reduction of the number of speech sounds

If, as Rudolf Steiner said, eurythmy should be visible speech, why then do an increasing number of eurythmists do so few sounds? I often ask myself this since, after years of being a stage artist, I have now become a member of the audience at eurythmy performances.

When I asked a few eurythmists, I was told that it is a further step in the development of eurythmy: everything is contained in a comprehensive word gesture so that making visible every single element of speech is no longer necessary.

For me it has always been so that Steiner intended eurythmy to make speech visible for physical eyes just as recitation or declamation is normally audible for physical ears, whether the latter is accompanied by eurythmy or spoken independently. It should be possible to write down exactly what one sees in a eurythmy performance in a kind of shorthand, and thereby understand what is being expressed. Indeed, Steiner made similar remarks in his introduction to 'The Twelve Moods' performance in 1915:

> It will gradually be understood that in this presentation the spoken word will be only one aspect contributing to the whole. Gradually it will be understood that if the movements are done in their fullness it will be possible to recognise from the movements what is being said, just as one can read the meaning in letters of the alphabet one is looking at. One need only have learned to read, and then gradually, when the whole system is developed, it will also be possible to read what is being presented here. One will be able to read not only in accordance with the letter, with the sound, but also in accordance with the meaning.[16]

An exception can be made when an actor is performing a monologue or taking part in dialogue, and this is accompanied by eurythmy. For instance, for the eurythmy accompanying the monologue spoken by Faust in the opening scene of *Faust* II, Steiner indicated that the chorus of elf beings should do very few speech sounds, especially in the first part of the monologue where they should do only one sound for every two lines:

> *The throb of life returns, with pulses beating*
> *Soft to ethereal dawn. O steadfast earth,*
>   during these lines form a slow L
>
> *True through the night, you waited for my greeting*
> *Breathing beneath my feet in glad new birth*[17]
>   an E slowly formed and then open

The whole should give the impression of a slow, expansive breathing, and the attention of the audience should not be diverted from the speaking Faust who accompanies his speech with a few expressive gestures.

Doing vowels and consonants without rushing

When one of the first eurythmists, Elisabeth Dolfuss (later Mrs Bauman), showed Rudolf Steiner a poem that she had worked on in 1915, he said that she was doing too few sounds. He told her to do all of the consonants as well as the vowels. When she said that it would look as though she were flailing about, Steiner replied that need not be the case if she practised everything thoroughly.

If a eurythmist performed all the vowels and consonants in a text, treating them equally and without the special quality that each sound has in the formation of a word, then hectic and agitated movement would indeed be unavoidable. But as is also the case with normal speaking or reading aloud, when performing eurythmy one should not monotonously chant the lines. Sounds should be *differentiated* according to their role in the structure of the word and in the transition from word to word. Bigger or smaller, slower or quicker eurythmy gestures modulate the performance just as an actor modulates their voice when reciting and declaiming. If it is not done in this way then eurythmy is no longer true, visible speech.

The quick tempo – appropriate for when the text is about small, delicate things, or when something is rushing past – can be expressed with small, fanciful movements of the hands or imaginative movements of the fingers, although these should not be in anyway arbitrary. Steiner told us that we should be careful what we do with our fingers and perform only those movements that are conscious and entirely controlled.

1919: On Tour

A new phase in the life of eurythmy began with the public performances in 1919. Rudolf Steiner always took part in the tours. He would give a short introductory lecture before every performance, standing on the stage in front of the closed curtain, introducing the audience to the origins, the artistic means, and the goals of eurythmy. Marie Steiner would recite the whole program from the box closest to the proscenium.

The response from audiences was mixed. In towns that had not been influenced by those hostile to our work, the reception was nearly always friendly and interested. People approached our art with open and enthusiastic hearts. But it also happened that we were followed by newspaper critics of a particularly scurrilous kind and by scandal-inciting groups. These were hired by our enemies in each place along with 'nervous' ladies who simulated hysterical laughter and convulsions during performances.

A strong, well-organised attack was scheduled for Frankfurt. Certain dubious characters distributed flyers at the entrance of the theatre, calling on attendees to join in the protest during the performance. The stagehands, who were on our side, warned us about the planned disruption and showed us the secret doors and exits. They were of the opinion that we were in danger of being attacked should we curtail the performance or if we carried on to the end and showed ourselves in the main entrance.

The first part of the program was delivered in an atmosphere of uneasy silence. No one dared to applaud, not even the few members of the anthroposophical society who were present. The protests came in the second part, when there was whistling, laughter and hysterical sighs. At times the noise was so great that Marie Steiner could no longer recite. She signalled to us that we should resist the attack and continue steadfastly to the end. Every time the noise dipped, Marie Steiner announced the title of the next piece in a strong, resounding voice and we appeared again, performing one piece after another with ever-increasing determination. I often remember with great joy our presentation of Goethe's poem 'The Yelping Dogs'. I performed the role of the poet who rides courageously through the world pursued by angry, barking dogs who threaten to tear him to pieces, while Marie Steiner recited the poem with an incredibly lively voice. The audience remained quiet for a few minutes, following the plot that Goethe had produced a hundred years before and which seemed to mirror what was happening at that moment.

At the end of the poem there was another loud protest, louder even than before. But from then on, one also heard applause and calls of 'Bravo!' too. A battle soon broke out between two factions in the audience, those demonstrating against us and those who supported us. The latter proved stronger and the group of whistling men and hysterical ladies were eventually escorted from the hall. The performance continued undisturbed to the end and was met with a loud applause from the sympathetic audience. Marie Steiner, who had endured the attacks so heroically, joined us on stage after the last item, which gave rise to exceptionally loud applause. We were all so proud of her and of ourselves, feeling that together we had fought a battle. The stagehands were also pleased for us, but nevertheless insisted on leading us through secret passages that took us out onto a dark side street.

Later that evening I returned to the house where I was lodging. The family I was staying with were critical of the anthroposophical movement and had not intended to come to the performance, but at the last minute they had informed me they had booked a box. After everything that had occurred that evening I did not know how I would be met. I hesitated at the door, wondering if I might not be better off finding a hotel for the night. But as it was late and I was tired, I rang the bell. The father of the family opened the door and greeted me with a radiant smile.

'You are true heroines!' he said. 'Did you hear how our box was the first to call out "Bravo!" and led the protest against those insolent conspirators? If all attacks on anthroposophy are like that, then from now on we wish to become friends of the movement. What a beautiful and noble art, and how heroic Marie Steiner and you eurythmists are!'

I heard later that this family had started studying spiritual science and attending lectures. Our enemies had miscalculated and rather than damaging the anthroposophical cause they had contributed to the success of it. Despite this victory, however, we were accompanied on our journey by this charming group of hecklers for quite a while.

Besides these protests, there were other difficulties that we had to overcome. Following a performance in Breslau* we were due to travel to Prague, but on the day of travel a railway strike broke out. At the border between Germany and Czechoslovakia, in the middle of the night, we had to leave the train laden with our luggage. A train guard with a lantern led this group of pilgrims through the snow and along the rough, dimly lit roads to the next village. When we got there the rooms in two of the inns were all taken, and everyone was asleep. In the last inn they were still celebrating carnival. The innkeeper took us up and showed us a large room. By the dim light of his candle we could see a few narrow beds, an old couch, and a few chairs around a table in the middle of the room.

Only three of us had a bed to ourselves that night. The others lay together on what was left. Leopold van der Pals made a bed on the couch, Jan Stuten, wrapped in his fur coat, crawled into a bed, and Louise Clason, who accompanied us on all our

---

* The city of Breslau was part of Germany until August 1945 when it became part of Poland. It is now called Wrocław.

journeys and who had a bad cold with a high fever, had a bed of her own. The rest of us made ourselves as comfortable as we could, which wasn't easy. The room was unheated and the temperature was twenty-four degrees below zero. We bundled ourselves up in coats and scarves, leaving only our eyes visible, and tried to sleep. This wasn't easy either. Almost immediately the mice began making noise, and several times during the night one of the eurythmists fell out of their narrow bed.

Early the next morning news came that the train to Prague would set off in half an hour. We jumped up and in the dim morning light looked around at the room that had sheltered us. It was filthy. The sheets on the beds had prints left by human hands and feet. The innkeeper explained that many soldiers had been billeted there and the room had not been cleaned since.

Thankfully, we made it to the station in time to catch the train and continued on our journey to Prague.

Marie Steiner was travelling with Mieta Pyle-Waller in a car belonging to Johanna von Keyserlingk. The car got stuck in the snow and had to be left behind. Fortunately, a baker's boy with a little sled came by. Marie Steiner was allowed to sit on it and, with feet dragging through the snow, was drawn to the next village. There they hired another vehicle that took them to the station to wait for the next train.

We had quite a few more misadventures on that tour and were glad when at last we returned to Dornach.

Through these experiences our strength increased. We also faced some resistance from the members of the society in the various town we visited. It happened on more than one occasion that members criticised the program and expressed misgivings over how it would be received. During and after a dress rehearsal it was frequently prophesied with great conviction that it would be a gigantic failure. Marie Steiner endured these moods with patience and astonishing calm. Then the performance would come and contrary to expectations the audience would show a willingness to go along with it, even an unexpected enthusiasm. Embarrassed and surprised, our pessimistic friends had to lay their mistrust aside and take the opportunity to examine their own judgment.

It was hardest for Marie Steiner when Rudolf Steiner could not accompany a eurythmy tour. During the above-mentioned tour, he was not able to be present. Now we had the opportunity to get to know Marie Steiner even better than before as a brave individual filled with a greatness of soul and an understanding of human nature. Her deep seriousness for the work was combined with humour and a refreshing joyfulness. She was for us an example of the right attitude towards the blows and fortunes of destiny, and of tireless self-sacrifice in the service of the spirit.

After one eurythmy performance, a gentleman from the audience burst into the box occupied by Marie Steiner. His manner was extremely insulting. He told her that he had not spent his money in order to see something so repellent, and that he would not tolerate such a non-art. Throughout his tirade, Marie Steiner listened calmly to the man. When he was finished she replied that she understood his aversion. Eurythmy is so dissimilar to anything that audiences are used to seeing in the dance world that it can take some time to become accustomed to it. Her composure disarmed the madman and he left the box without another word. It turned out that he was an unemployed actor from Salzburg, although whether he had been hired to insult Marie Steiner or was just giving vent to his own personal frustrations wasn't clear.

Appreciative and well-intentioned reviews were not allowed to appear. When submitting their reviews, reporters had to indicate whether they were 'pro' or 'contra'. Those who wrote 'pro' were dismissed with the comment that only 'contra' would be accepted. It belongs to the destiny of a new and significant impulse, especially in the realm of the spirit, to walk a path of thorns and tread the modern way of the martyr.

During these tours we got to know the many members of the society who looked after us. They arranged social gatherings and showed us the local sights. But most touching of all was the willingness with which they shared their meagre food. This was the post-war period and great need and deprivation were everywhere. Through this love and great generosity of spirit a beautiful bond was created between us.

Eurythmy lessons were introduced in many towns as a result of these tours.

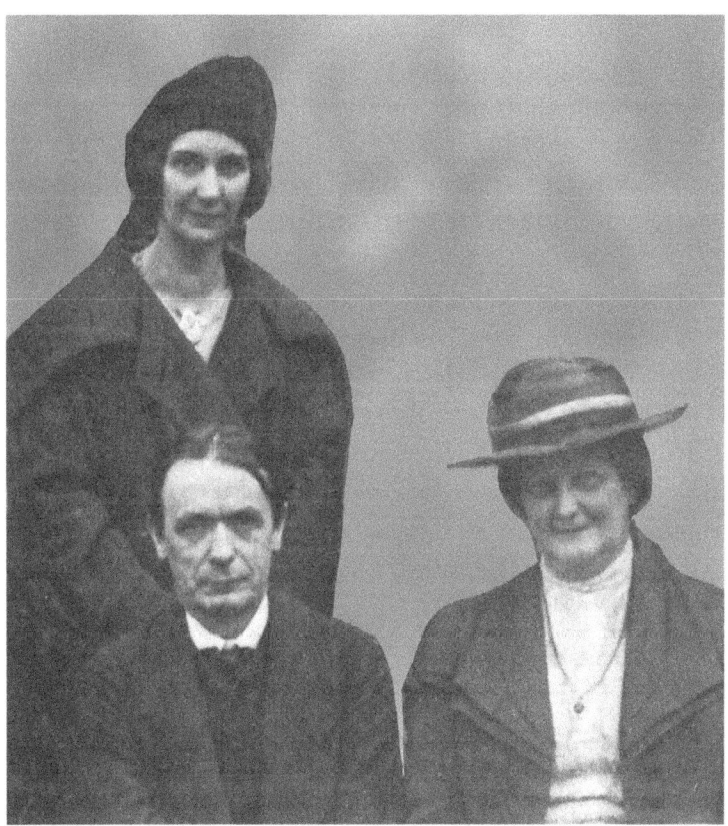

Detail from a group photograph taken in Oxford in 1922 showing Rudolf and Marie Steiner with Tatiana Kisseleff standing behind.

1919–24:
In the House of the Word

On the stage of the Goetheanum

Already in the first years of our work in the Carpenter's Shop, coloured electric footlights were fixed to the stage and Rudolf Steiner began developing the art of lighting in connection with eurythmy. This reached a particular perfection in the first Goetheanum, where our eurythmy performances took place after it opened in 1920.

It is difficult to describe the beauty of the picture that was revealed to the audience when the curtain opened on the stage of the Goetheanum for the first time. It was a unique and incomparable setting. Here our art of eurythmy was united in a profoundly harmonious way with the paintings of the cupola and the forms of the architraves, capitals and pillars. The eurythmists, especially in the group pieces, appeared as if winged, with their wafting coloured veils that flowed over their light and dark dresses as they moved in energetic waves through the richly differentiated, spiritually lawful dances. All was wonderfully interwoven with coloured light streaming through the glass windows. It is hard to convey for those who were not there to experience it the wealth of creative expression that arose through the introduction of this art into the ambience of that building.

In this artistic environment Marie Steiner recited for eurythmy for the next three years. She was the creator of this new art of speech formation, and remains, in my view, the greatest master in all areas of language: whether in the sublime and majestic mode or the intimate inwardness of soul, in dramatic characterisation or the exhilarating humoresques. I am incredibly grateful that it was my destiny to be carried by Marie Steiner's recitations in the many poems I performed in the Carpenter's Shop and on stage in the Goetheanum. I know that the other eurythmists who shared the good fortune of being inspired by Marie Steiner also feel the same gratitude in their hearts. She recited for one and all, regardless of the burden, repeating single lines a number of times until the movement on the stage could unite with the spoken word. Her suggestions and corrections, her invaluable remarks and conversations, brought out the best in those eurythmists with whom she worked. Next to Rudolf Steiner, we owe a great deal of what is pure and innocent in eurythmy to Marie Steiner.

In her introduction to *Speech and Drama*, Marie Steiner speaks about 'the healing and magic forces of the word, the waves of spirituality which pour out from it'. She continues, 'Speech is flowing movement carried by an inner music in colourful, magical images and sculptural forms.'[1] Not only did Marie Steiner say that, but she also lived it, and because she did, the art of eurythmy was able to develop. She worked tirelessly in the realm of speech – surrounded by artists who had come to Dornach, dissatisfied, full of questions, and asking her for guidance – so that, step by step, she might lead the way to the lofty goal of spiritualising and ensouling the word.

Rudolf Steiner often said that the building of the Goetheanum was just a feeble beginning, a first step towards the creation of an artform able to reveal the special artistic life that seeks to manifest in our time.

> The risk had to be taken to lead over from the more mathematical-dynamic style to the organic-living style. It may be as imperfect as it is possible to be today, but a beginning had to be made.[2]

In a lecture he gave on December 29, 1914, he said that eurythmy is necessary for our time and that it had to enter into human evolution, but this should not give rise to arrogance among eurythmists. In the same lecture, Steiner relates the different artforms to the various members of the human being: for example, he connects architecture with the physical body, sculpture with the etheric body, painting with the astral body, music with the ego, and poetry with the Spirt-self, which humanity is not destined to receive in its fullness until a future epoch of Earth evolution. He connects the art of eurythmy with a still higher member of the human being, the Life Spirit. Of this connection, he says:

> At the moment this is something that will only reach a certain degree of perfection in the very distant future ... what we can say in this domain is like the babbling of a child when compared with the later perfection of speech.[3]

I consider these remarks by Steiner about the building of the Goetheanum and the art of eurythmy to be immensely important. He speaks about taking a risk and of something incomplete when drawing people's attention to Goethean art, and when referring to the young art of eurythmy he says it will only reach a certain degree of perfection in the very far future.

Steiner liked to say, 'Test yourself, student, practise with great diligence!' He said we should make this our motto and that it should be written, not only in every eurythmist's diary or notebook, but above all in their hearts, so that it becomes an underlying mood. It reminds us that we are only at the beginning of this new artform and it can prevent us from falling prey to the arrogance Steiner warned against in his lecture. After all, are we not all only students of eurythmy, as we were students of spiritual science and still are today?

In her introduction to *Speech and Drama*, Marie Steiner writes how Rudolf Steiner brought about the synthesis of the arts in the building of the Goetheanum itself, as well as describing in a beautiful way the general synthesis between art, science, and religion that he achieved:

> The building stood there like the human being, the human being as a building. The coming into being of the world, the coming into being and activity of human beings, the deeds of the gods were inscribed into it, were revealed in the weaving colour of the cupola, in the organic growth of the columns and architrave motifs, in the shapes in the windows. Sculpture and painting went beyond themselves, overcame the line and went over into movement. Colour created the forms out of itself, out of its own creative soul nature. In the newly blossoming art of eurythmy, musical tones and speech became movement and stepped into visibility through the instrument of the human being. So having now become visible, the creative forces of speech worked back onto the other arts in an enlivening way, kindling a spiritual creative fire. The inner tone residing inwardly could grasp the tone produced in the air, spiritualise it, and lift it into higher spheres. Rudolf Steiner had named it the House of the Word. All *arts* found a home there and *science* and *mystery wisdom*. The synthesis of art, science and religion was accomplished again.[4]

The eurythmy figures

In December 1922, the art of eurythmy received a strong new impulse. It was announced that Steiner would give a lecture in the Carpenter's Shop. On the stage, to the right and left of the speaker's podium, two high structures were placed with something hidden behind a paper covering. During the lecture, Steiner spoke about the mediums of the various arts, such as sculpture, dramatic art, declamation. Proceeding to eurythmy, he pointed out that this art expresses itself through the *movement, feeling* and *character* of the human being. In other words, the whole human being is the medium through which the art of eurythmy expresses itself.

At the end of the lecture Steiner removed the paper covering between the two high structures, and we saw a row of coloured wooden figures. They represented the sounds of the alphabet and the gestures of the soul moods. Each one depicted all three elements that Steiner had spoken about in the lecture: movement, feeling, and character, in three different colours.

'These figures were made to help those who want to practise and perfect themselves in the art of eurythmy,' Steiner said. 'They were suggested by Edith Maryon, who made them according to my indications.'

For those who loved eurythmy, that was a joyful, celebratory moment.

New Year's Eve, 1922

During the Christmas week of 1922, festive performances were held in the Goetheanum. On New Year's Eve, the 'Prologue in Heaven' (*Faust: Part One*) was performed in the uniquely beautiful setting of the small cupola, and then later, among other poems, Vladimir Solovyov's 'The New Year Also Always Brings New Graves'.

That evening Steiner gave one of his most powerful lectures. He spoke of humanity's responsibility for the destiny of the earth, and about the possibility of a cosmic *cultus* for human beings of the present day. He also spoke about the possibility of communicating spiritually with divine beings through independent, creative thoughts, if only human beings would make real what is present in their will. Out of the necessary continuous dying of the earthly world, new life will emerge next to the 'new graves' mentioned in Solovyov's poem speaks; 'new cradles' will be erected, and the earth will receive seeds for the future if human beings decide to be active and make real the renewal of the earth in the world-historical New Year.[5]

Shortly after the end of the lecture the fire in the Goetheanum broke out. During the course of that night the Goetheanum was sacrificed to the flames.

In the aftermath of the fire, we continued our eurythmy work in the Carpenter's Shop. A wealth of new forms for tone and speech eurythmy were given to us during this time, including forms for poems in different languages along with indications for the treatment of the sounds in these languages (see p. 157, Eurythmy in other languages).

With the greatest devotion and enthusiasm, Marie Steiner dedicated herself to expressing the poetic style of each folk in the recitations that accompanied our eurythmy performances. Her deep, living connection to most of the European languages, and her encompassing knowledge of world literature, astounded us all. Marie Steiner's ability to perceive the soul and spirit of the poetry of different epochs connected with her creative ability to express the spiritual content of each poetical work in a perfected manner of speaking. French, English, Italian, Russian, Dutch, and other poems appeared successively in our eurythmy programs; the voices of many nations were heard. This artistic ability of Marie Steiner's had a great social effect too. It provided an impulse towards understanding one another, creating bonds between the representatives of almost twenty nationalities who, through the manifold paths of destiny, found themselves in Dornach in those years.

The Goetheanum as the 'House of the Word'

Rudolf Steiner once said of the first Goetheanum that it was 'the beginning of an attempt', an 'incomplete first step', and while this uniquely beautiful work of architecture may have fallen short of its creator's intentions, those who were graced by destiny to enter this place – especially the small group of people who were active within it – received into their souls a wealth of spiritual impulses. They were allowed to witness the sunrise of a completely new era in artistic life that stood as a polar opposite to the gloominess of the materialistic culture of the day.

This incredible building may have lasted only a short while, but spiritually it lives on, not only in the memory of those few who were active there, but also in every soul that does not close itself off from its spiritual effects. It continues to live as light and warmth that works to bring about spiritual awakening. Because it sprang out of love for the spirit and was built with enthusiasm, this building sheltered within its material the noblest sacrificial substance, which does not perish even when the substance is destroyed.[6]

What the best of those individuals of the nineteenth century who sought for true spiritual values longed for – what Goethe, Schiller, Wagner and others dimly sensed – was fulfilled through the bringer of anthroposophical spiritual science and art. Through Rudolf Steiner, the future ideal, the reconciliation of the visual and musical arts, became a reality in the Goetheanum. Rudolf Steiner spoke about his attempt to bring the architectural forms into 'musical flux' in the Goetheanum, and he said that penetration

> ...of the fine arts and their forms by musical moods has to be the fundamental ideal of the art of the future ... Architecture and sculpture of the future will be more musical than they were in the past. That will be the essential thing.[7]

And this future came into being in this building. All that was achieved by Rudolf Steiner personally or through others under his direction – in architecture, sculpture, painting, coloured glass windows – took on musically flowing form and brought the soul out into the widths of the cosmos. Everything was a speech organ in the building that Steiner called the House of the Word.

Alongside the building of the Goetheanum, the art of eurythmy also grew. In many lectures about eurythmy, Steiner juxtaposed the resting forms of the sculptor with the moving forms of eurythmy, describing it as moving sculpture expressed in the speaking of the soul through the movement of the human being – a 'visible speech' or a 'visible singing'. Through this art of movement is given to us the means to fulfil the task of our time: to bring out the hidden cosmic forces that are inwardly concentrated in the microcosmic human being and give them back to the world. Rudolf Steiner says,

With very few exceptions, eurythmy was accompanied by recitation and declamation. The silent introductions, where there was no text to be recited, often had musical accompaniment, which the musicians in Dornach composed, stimulated by the new art and Rudolf Steiner's indications.

Marie Steiner's great spiritual deed was the ensouling of speech: her creative spirit allowed the living soul-filled speech of past ages to be resurrected. From the very beginning, Marie Steiner was intensively connected with eurythmy and guided the work of eurythmy in Dornach and Germany. Reciting and declaiming for all rehearsals and performances herself, she completely accomplished the spiritual regeneration of the withered art of speech. By bringing back the artistic element of speech, the sculptural, imaginative and musical qualities, she brought back to life the hidden eurythmy in speech and developed a method for the art of speech formation. Through Marie Steiner, this rescued, ensouled and spiritually appropriate speaking could appear as an independent art next to eurythmy. At the beginning, she had attempted to recite and do eurythmy simultaneously, performing the Earth Spirit in *Faust* and the character of Felicia Balde in one of Rudolf Steiner's Mystery Dramas. But Marie Steiner immediately recognised that this was not feasible and divided these artistic activities between the speaker and the eurythmist. Rudolf Steiner left her alone in her search and wrestling with this problem, but expressed himself completely in agreement with her solution. From that point onwards, the relationship between the arts of eurythmy, recitation and music was realised in what Rudolf Steiner called 'the orchestral working together' of the different elements. The 'overburdening of human activity through simultaneous eurythmy and speaking' was prevented in this way.

Intense work was also being done in the area of dramatic art. The *Speech and Drama* course held by Rudolf and Marie Steiner in 1924 was the result of their creative working together over many years in the realm of the art of the word. In her article 'The Mysteries of the Word', Marie Steiner reminds us of this course and brings significant considerations about the mysteries of the word. She speaks of the necessity of 'transforming oneself through ceaseless work on the revelations of the word'.[8] She portrays eurythmy as a bridge, providing us with the means to grasp the forces that connect to the supersensible in a real way. These forces show the artist the path to overcoming what belongs to the merely reasoning mind because they have nothing to do with mental constructs. Rather, eurythmy reaches deeply into life and into the lawfulness of the cosmos.

Rudolf Steiner's hope that eurythmy would have a health-giving, fructifying effect on the other arts was also fulfilled. Eurythmy opened up new possibilities of expression in music and following eurythmical principles of colour eurythmy, the lighting and costume arts could be elevated beyond the subjective and arbitrary quality of the times. Through the connection of eurythmy with drama, the problem of presenting the interplay between the supersensible and earthly events was also solved.

***

For three years, this unique and wonderful building, the Goetheanum, revealed the deepest mysteries of the world and human development through the language of form and colour, through the spoken word and the silent speech of eurythmy. Through the synthesis of the arts, and then an even more all-embracing synthesis of art, science, and religion, the visitor was able to experience the rising spiritual light in the midst of the darkness of our materialistic world. After the fire, this 'outer representation of the anthroposophical spiritual stream' was no longer physically there. Only the wooden sculpture, the Group or the Representative of Humanity, depicting the higher Christ-permeated human nature placed between its two adversaries, has been left to us by destiny. It introduces the meaning of the Earth to the human being and points toward the aim of Earth evolution and the task of humanity. These three forces carved out of wood, are active in the human being. The search for the spiritual world in oneself can lead, on the one hand, to a striving for personal perfection and a turning away from the outer world, or to its opposite pole, living a purely materialistic life and thereby losing oneself in the world. One finds the balance when one can unite oneself in the right way with the Christ-impulse.

The polarity of these two principles occupied Goethe a great deal during his long life of spiritual searching, and in *Faust* he strove for a synthesis of both paths. But it was only through Rudolf Steiner that this problem was consciously and fully solved. In the realm of art this came about especially through the four Mystery Dramas in which Steiner's spiritual knowledge and esoteric teaching are realised dramatically.

The first Goetheanum was built mainly with the Mystery Dramas in mind; due to their essential nature and style it was felt that a suitable setting was needed. At the suggestion of a number of members in the Anthroposophical Society, especially those who organised the Mystery Drama festivals and the following lecture cycles by Steiner in Munich, the name Johannesbau (Johannes Building) was chosen for this building. This had to do with one of the main characters of the Mystery Dramas, Johannes Thomasius. It was originally planned to build it in Munich but that was not possible. The first initiative to build a 'temple' for Rudolf Steiner's work came in 1908 from Mieta Waller (late Mieta Pyle-Waller) who also donated the first 'building stone'. She was the first to portray Johannes Thomasius between 1910–13.

The Mystery Dramas present the soul-spiritual development of a group of people and the opposition they experience from certain spiritual forces when crossing the threshold to the spiritual world. On the one hand there are the ahrimanic powers who want to bind human beings to a purely physical and mechanical existence. On the other, there are the luciferic powers who want to alienate human beings from their earthly tasks and entice them towards an abstract spiritual world. It has already been mentioned that the first eurythmy performance given in Munich in 1912, was the dance of the luciferic and ahrimanic thought-beings from the sixth scene of the Mystery Drama *The Guardian of the Threshold* (see p. 17).

The same motif presented in the wooden sculpture was also painted by Rudolf Steiner on the small cupola, the dome above the stage of the building. In this painting, and especially in the magnificent sculpture carved by Steiner himself, the 'content and substance of the anthroposophical movement of the present day and future' came to expression.

The sculpture was meant to have stood at the most important place in the building: on the level of the stage. This was portrayed in a picture made by the artist William Scott Pyle. This never came to pass unfortunately because of the fire that destroyed the building on New Year's Eve 1922. Later, the wooden sculpture was moved from Rudolf Steiner's studio in the Carpenter's Shop where he had been working on it, over to a side room in the second Goetheanum.

The beginning of eurythmy training

At the beginning of 1924, the Eurythmy School in Dornach was officially founded with three classes 'under the direction of Tatiana Kisseleff', together with a few stage artists as the first teachers. In 1925 the fourth class was added. Introductory courses had existed since 1916, training courses now followed.

In February, 1924, Rudolf Steiner gave a comprehensive course on tone eurythmy. This was a new chapter added to the course first given in 1915, and one that enriched music eurythmy with mighty impulses. In the summer, a new speech eurythmy course was given in a large auditorium to a large audience of eurythmists, actors and other co-workers living in and around Dornach and from elsewhere. The course lasted from June 24 until July 12 and consisted of fifteen lectures that presented a wealth of material and the deepest impulses for further work. These lectures later appeared in print in 1927 under the title *Eurythmy as Visible Speech*. It included an introduction by Marie Steiner and a series of excerpts from introductory talks Steiner had given before eurythmy performances. The lecture cycle on tone eurythmy also appeared in print in 1927 under the title *Eurythmy as Visible Singing*.[9]

If one wanted to describe all that had taken place and been worked out through eurythmy during the first fourteen years at the Goetheanum, one would need to add much more. Here I have only been able to describe some special features of this important period of time. In its first seven years eurythmy developed quickly and joyously under the immediate guidance of its creators, Rudolf and Marie Steiner. The next seven-year period was concerned with journeying through the European world and bringing the healing forces inherent in eurythmy wherever it was possible. This occurred in a kind of spiralling motion outwards before returning back to the centre, to the Goetheanum, where Rudolf Steiner would provide us with new impulses before we resumed our journeying.

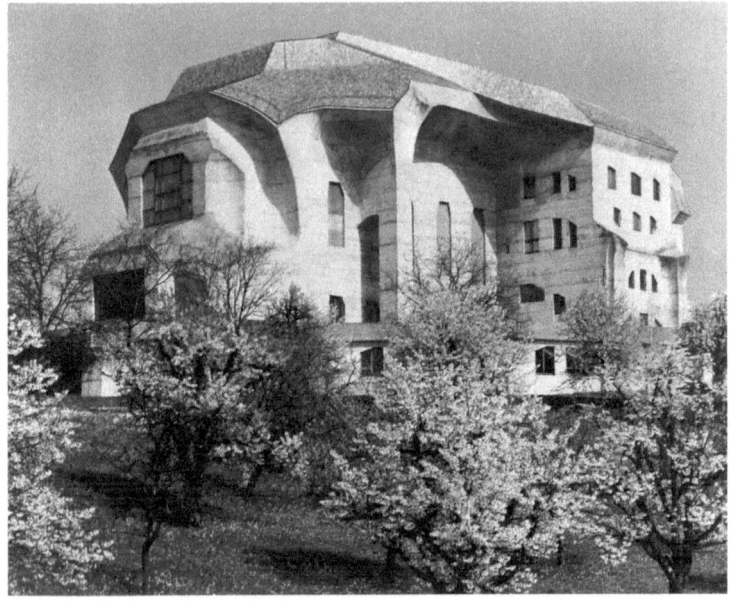

The Goetheanum, School for Spiritual Science in Dornach, Switzerland, re-opened 1928.

These powerful impulses were also a pledge for the continued development of eurythmy on earth, both in the present and on into the distant future. When we show ourselves worthy of the trust that has been placed in us, then what has been given will raise humanity to a higher level. Eurythmy, the original art of movement raised to present day consciousness, will lead us forwards, step by step, toward the exalted goal: the resurrection of the Word in human beings.

1924–27:
Rudolf Steiner's Death –
A Turning Point in My Life

In its first decade eurythmy was able to develop in the spiritual light that streamed so abundantly from its source and from which we could draw upon directly. During that time I experienced the fulfilment of all the longing and endeavour that had marked my early years.

I had always been interested in the art of movement, but I found little to satisfy me in the various artistic dance performances I experienced. Even Isadora Duncan's approach to dance, which gifted students in Russia followed, left me unsatisfied. I had lived in Moscow in a studio which was above a dance school belonging to a successor of Duncan. I heard the music and the noise coming from the studio, and I saw the large numbers of students that went in and out from morning until evening, but I had no wish to join them. I did not want to become a barefoot dancer dressed in some sort of Greek costume.

Around this time, 1909–10, I began to search for a new form of dance. Once, while reading a religious-philosophical work by Vladimir Solovyov, I experienced the desire to move rhythmically. I put the book aside and began to dance. The movements I made gave me great pleasure, except that I did not know what to do with my arms; they always stayed in the same upwards chalice-like gesture. I felt like an empty vessel, my soul suspended in a mood of expectation. I did not want to do arabesque-like movements or fleeting mime-like gestures as

I had seen some dancers do. I visited dancers' private studios and was also allowed to visit a dance rehearsal in the practice studio of a theatre, but I did not want to enrol as a student because I was repelled by the movements of the arms and hands that I saw everywhere.

Then when I saw eurythmy for the first time, very imperfectly done, I knew immediately that I had found what I had sensed must exist, and what I had always longed for: the fulfilment of my deep yearning for beautiful, meaningful arm movement.

At the same time, I read the lecture cycle that Rudolf Steiner had given in Kassel called *The Gospel of St. John and Its Relation to the Other Gospels*. In the eighth lecture he speaks about Solovyov's philosophical system:

> But those who do not have spiritual science achieve no more than an empty conceptual form. This is the case also in the profound thinker Solovyov. His philosophical systems resemble vessels for containing concepts; and what must be poured into them is something they indeed crave and for which they form the moulds ... and this can come only out of the anthroposophical current. It will fill the moulds with that living water which is the revelation of facts concerning the spiritual world ... This is what the spiritual-scientific world outlook will offer these finest minds, who already today show that they need it, and whose tragedy lies in their not having been able to obtain it. We can say of such minds that they positively yearn for anthroposophy. But they have not been able to find it. It is the task of the anthroposophical movement to pour into these vessels, prepared by such minds, all that can contribute to clear, distinct, true conceptions of the most significant events, such as the Christ even and the Mystery of Golgotha.[1]

This series of lectures was held in 1909, around the same time that I danced with my arms raised in the gesture of a chalice having just read a lecture by Solovyov.

I will now describe my further efforts and observations with eurythmy as I worked through the invaluable gift of anthroposophy. This continued in Dornach for a while before I took what had been cultivated at the Goetheanum to another place.

But first, I would like to give an account of specific problems and particular considerations concerning the future development of eurythmy.

I return to the years 1924–25. From September 1924, Rudolf Steiner was ill in bed, which he had moved to the Carpenter's Shop. In spite of this, he continued to send us forms for eurythmy with various indications for costumes, lighting, and so on. These included forms for a few poems by Albert Steffen, as well as the forms for the Michael Verse, 'Springing from Powers of the Sun' (we performed the verse for the first time only after his death at Easter, 1925).

Then came March 30, 1925, followed by the celebration of that great mystery in the Carpenter's Shop. We saw Rudolf Steiner for the last time on the stage surrounded by a sea of flowers. For this reason, this first primitive stage of the Goetheanum is for me the most unique, exalted, most holy of all stages. It speaks a deeply significant and mysterious language. It is unceasingly dear to me and will remain so forever.

Rudolf Steiner was no longer physically present; the wellspring that had given us life and healing for so many years had withdrawn. But for those who have found each other in the spirit there is no separation; this we knew from Steiner for he spoke to us about it often.

Now it was up to us to nurture what he had left us, to care for the eurythmy he had given us, and to grow with it so that in the future we might make his gift our own. He had given us so much, especially in his last years, and we drew strength for further life and work from his words. He had placed before us a high goal: to recreate through movement the heavenly archetype of the human being. On this subject he had said:

> If a person feels that here on earth they do not fulfil what lies in their *archetype*, with its abode in the heavens, then there arises in such a person an artistic longing for some outer image of that *archetype*. Whereupon they can gain the power to become an instrument for bringing to expression the true relationship of the human being to the world by becoming a eurythmist.[2]

That was the task he placed before us, the path he allowed us to tread. It is a long path and a holy task and represents more than can be achieved in a single lifetime. This was only a beginning for us, the first step that we were able to take.

We held a eurythmy celebration for Rudolf Steiner. And then, as had to be, we were left to make our own compositions in speech and tone eurythmy. Next to Steiner's wonderful artistic forms and indications, ours were imperfect attempts, rather like a helpless babble. Marie Steiner allowed us to search and feel our way through them, putting together programs for the performances and become more independent. She was patient and encouraging, and she enjoyed our efforts.

In the following years she travelled a great deal and was often away for a long time. Sometimes she took part of the eurythmy group with her in order to give eurythmy performances in various places.

In August 1925, there was a week of practical work at the Goetheanum for eurythmy teachers. Nearly fifty teachers came together for this work, most of them from Germany. The lessons, which I gave with the help of Erika Klug-Schilbach, and the practice sessions for the teachers took place in a large tent that had been erected on the grounds of the

Goetheanum near to where the observatory now stands. The work proceeded in a beautiful, harmonious manner. In the hours between the lessons and practices, we rested on the grass under the summer skies.

Marie Steiner visited us once toward the end of the course. Happy and delighted at the sight of moving, colourful forms in this natural setting, she suggested we give a eurythmy teachers' performance with the tent as a stage and with those lounging in the meadow as audience. Unfortunately, it rained on the day of the performance. At the last minute we had to reorganise a reduced program and give two performances on the small stage in the Carpenter's Shop. Nevertheless, over twenty eurythmists participated. The Pater Noster, with Steiner's indications, was also performed for the first time with a large group of teachers.

Between 1925 and 1926 I worked mainly with the new generation of eurythmists on the courses first given by Steiner in 1915 and 1924. I also taught the actors who had come to Rudolf and Marie Steiner from various parts of Germany in the summer of 1924, with their many questions and problems. In September of that same year a course in speech formation and dramatic art was held. In a lecture from the dramatic course, Steiner says that the art of eurythmy is closely related to today's stage art:

> We have to consider that this art of eurythmy will be entirely one with today's stage art in the future, as we must already acknowledge that it is in an outward way; the art of acting will in the future consider eurythmy as something that simply belongs to it.

In the eleventh lecture he speaks about how the actor will make use of eurythmy, not directly with their performance continually flowing into eurythmy, but indirectly:

> For what have we in eurythmy? In eurythmy we
> have the full, the macrocosmic gesture for vowel
> and consonant ... fill yourself with the ghost of the
> eurythmic form, with its mirrored reflection, and
> while still feeling the form there within you, intone.
> In this way you will come to speak your vowels and
> consonants in their purity.[3]

In her introductory words to this course, Marie Steiner says that in eurythmy, Steiner 'gave a new art that has power in it to animate and fructify all the other arts'.[4]

My memories of working with these enthusiastic, devoted young artists are among the most beautiful of that period. Many of them lived in primitive, barrack-like huts behind the bushes on the way from the canteen to the Goetheanum. The people from the village called this little camp 'the poor man's village.' It was cold in winter, hot in summer, and without any conveniences. For all that, this group of young people found themselves at the wellspring of a new artistic life that centred around Marie Steiner; they were her first pupils, her future group of actors.

The founding of this actors' group took place on September 29, 1924, Michaelmas Day. They were called Thespians after Thespis, born on the Attic island of Icaria in the sixth century BC. According to Aristotle, Thespis was the first person to appear on stage as an actor playing a character rather than themselves. He was the creator of tragic drama and is also acknowledged as the creator of the dances of the chorus. He added the dithyrambic choral singing of the stories and orchestral mime performances of the Dionysian myths to the Dionysian festivals. He also seems to have invented theatrical touring. In his *Ars Poetica*, Horace mentions that Thespis travelled around with his props and costumes and masks in a horse-drawn wagon. Marie Steiner suggested the name of the group in view of the fact that drama had arisen out of the Mysteries, and that human beings should seek to bring drama back to its source. Rudolf Steiner had agreed.

At that time we had quite a number of men who practised eurythmy with great devotion and enthusiasm. Thanks to their dramatic gifts and their abilities to express different characters, it was possible to bring variety into our eurythmy performances. I worked with these men on different ways of walking, how to hold their heads and position their bodies, as well as the differentiated ways of moving their arms in order to express the temperaments. When a poem had been worked out, we showed it to Marie Steiner who gave us advice and encouragement.

When she returned from her travels, Marie Steiner told us of her experiences in the countries she had visited, and the many people she met who were striving for the spirit but who did not have the possibility of coming to Dornach. Sometimes she would turn to a eurythmist and ask them if they would be willing to go to some town or other in order to work more thoroughly with the people there on cultivating eurythmy. But the eurythmists to whom she spoke usually said that they were not willing to leave Dornach to work in the world outside.

By the end of 1926, however, the decision had ripened in me to share what I had learned of eurythmy and anthroposophy over the last fifteen years with those living far away, people who either knew nothing about the Goetheanum or who were unable to come to Dornach. It was not an easy decision to leave. The roots that connected me to this place went deep; the Goetheanum was my home, and the people who lived in Dornach had become my family. Nevertheless I was able to overcome the somewhat egotistical way of thinking that tempted me to continue my work in Dornach, and although I experienced many difficulties in the years that followed, I never regretted my decision to leave. A new chapter in my life began at that moment.

Before I relate what happened to me after I left Dornach, I would like to consider the path described by the life of human beings through the zodiac while they are still on earth.

In 1915, after we had received the division of the twelve consonants in the zodiac and performed 'The Twelve Moods' for the first time, Rudolf Steiner said to me that every poem could be done in this way, that any cyclical development, for example the course of the life of a person, could be presented in eurythmy. To illustrate this he gave two possible situations in the destiny of a person. Let us assume a law student has passed their last exam, they have achieved the goal they were set. In this case one would place the eurythmy forms in the region of Leo. Or perhaps the student has failed instead, and thereby bitterly disappointed the hopes of their parents. The whole episode would then be done in the region of Scorpio. That does not mean, Steiner added, that the student has failed absolutely. It could also be that the student leaves their homeland after the fiasco they suffered because their parents and other people do not want to have anything more to do with him. They go, let us say, to America and apply themselves to all sorts of things. Then one day they produce a drawing that pleases a connoisseur. The connoisseur commissions them and the failed law student ends up becoming a successful and significant artist.

In the years after 1915, I was always looking for poems that described the course of life in order to perform them in this way, but I was never able to work out a whole biography. During the last eurythmy course in 1924, Steiner once again spoke about the zodiac in connection with eurythmy. He placed twelve eurythmists in a circle on the stage. Each one had to respond to a specific consonant and received indications from Steiner on how the consonant in question emerged out of the position and gesture of the arms and the head preceding it. I had to do Cancer, to which the sound F is allocated. According to Steiner's indication, the mood of Cancer is the 'impulse toward deeds'. In an earlier lecture Steiner had said that in the constellation of Cancer one period of development ends and a new one begins.

Now it appeared to be the case that I had entered the region of Cancer in the course of my life and received its impulse to bring about a change in my destiny. As early as 1912 I had known that it belonged to my future tasks to bring spiritual science to the Russians. Steiner had spoken about this to me a few times. Already during our first conversation in Munich, in 1912, he had placed this task before me. At that time I was shocked to hear him speak to me of this. After all the disasters that I had experienced in Russia so recently, after all the tribulations of searching for the spiritual source that I had now found, he seemed to be saying I would have to return to Russia. At the time I felt it was beyond my capacities. I expressed my concerns to Steiner, but he reassured me by outlining the following plan: I could spend part of the year in the centre of the anthroposophical movement, then take what I had received from spiritual science to Russia for the remaining part, but always I would return to the source. I was completely in agreement with this plan for my life and work. Unfortunately, I could not realise it in the following years. The war and then the revolution in Russia, prevented me from undertaking these journeys.

In December 1918, Rudolf Steiner spoke to me for the last time about the urgent necessity that the Russian people take up anthroposophy as quickly as possible. I was called to the studio where he was working on the Group – the sculpture of The Representative of Man, Lucifer, and Ahriman that was to stand in the Goetheanum – and found Rudolf and Marie Steiner talking about the situation in Russia at that time. The anthroposophist Andrei Belyi, a well-known and talented Russian author, had with other significant artists successfully performed their works in a well-heated venue in a distinguished hotel. They had met with great success and overall had been treated well. Heating and good food were rare exceptions in that time of cold, need, and extreme hunger in Russia. Steiner voiced his opinion that in spite of its high status, this venue was not the right setting in which to introduce the art of eurythmy to the public and that under these circumstances there was no question of me travelling to Russia.

Steiner was very worried about how disastrous it would be if anthroposophy were not introduced to the Russian people in the next ten years. If this were not to happen, it would be a long time before the opportunity arose again. In the following years I frequently asked myself how and when I would fulfil the task Steiner had given me concerning the people of Russia, in whom there lies the seed of a future spirituality.

Eight years went by. Then, in the autumn of 1926, I spoke with Marie Steiner about the possibility of this work. She mentioned three large cities: Prague, Warsaw and Paris. These were the main centres of Russian emigration. Although Warsaw was my place of birth, I decided on Paris. During my student days at the University of Lausanne, where I received my diploma in Social Science and Law, I had also spent time in Paris and attended the University there. I had and also worked in the field of Experimental Psychology at the psychiatric hospital in Villejuif. As someone from the east, I needed to find a balance in the west. And so, in January 1927, I left Dornach and moved to Paris.

1927–39: Paris – Studio rue Huyghens and the École Rudolf Steiner

A new life began for me that was in many ways very different from the one I had led in Dornach. It began promisingly enough. In Paris I found people who were striving after the spirit, and who responded with delight when I told them about the 'wonder of Dornach' as they called it: a place where people from all warring nations had come together to carry out Rudolf Steiner's healing work while hate and destruction raged outside.

My work was introduced with a eurythmy performance in which two eurythmists from Dornach also took part. After this first performance in French and Russian, another followed for a smaller circle of invited Russians. Among them was the ex-Grand Duke Alexander Mikhailovich, former advisor and brother-in-law to Tsar Nicholas II. After the performance he told me he was pleased to see people doing movements that certain spiritual beings use when manifesting themselves in their speech.

A few days after this performance, which aroused great interest, I was informed that I was not permitted to stay in Paris. Deeply concerned, I spoke about this with Paul Coroze, the husband of eurythmist Simone Rihouët-Coroze. He listened to me with a mysterious smile, then took me to see the Chief of Police. Mr Coroze spoke briefly to him about my situation. To my great astonishment the Chief of Police expressed his admiration for the 'magnificent artistic achievement' he had seen two days ago in the studio. Mr Coroze had had the brilliant idea of inviting this high-ranking official to our performance, and now the Chief of Police wanted to know what I thought the effect of this spiritual art would be on the greater Parisian public. Did I think it would be received by large numbers of people, with many of them perhaps learning eurythmy for themselves? I answered honestly that I thought it would appeal to only a relatively small group of people. He thought that was quite right, that was probably how it would be, and it was good to have no illusions on the matter. We would have to satisfy ourselves with a 'small, elite group', as the majority of Parisians enjoyed quite another kind of dance.

'If you still want to work in spite of this,' he said, 'I will be happy to give you a permit to stay for the period of time allowed by law.'

The Chief of Police then left me alone in his office while he went with Mr Coroze into another room to arrange the paperwork.

The remarkably accommodating and understanding attitude of this Chief of Police made me think about another high official in Paris who plays such an important part in the poem 'The Crocodile, or the Battle between Good and Evil' by Saint-Martin. It is a poem in the epic-magical style, half satirical, half allegorical, and composed of 102 'songs'. It describes how the Crocodile, a servant of the Dragon, the spirit of matter, takes over Paris, and how the society of the spiritually free fight backs and eventually triumphs over them. The victory owes a great deal to the fact that the safety of the city has been entrusted to a magistrate called Sédir, who enjoys the respect of the population because of his dignity and fairness, and because he is strongly drawn to the most elevated religious truths. After the victory he is accepted into the society of the spiritually free.

I received a permit for residency and assurance from the Chief of Police said I could turn to him for help if I ever experienced problems with the police during the course of my activity in Paris. A few months later he helped me with a visa for a short visit to Dornach. Mr Coroze was radiant on our return journey and spoke about our battle with crocodiles and the victory we had achieved. I congratulated him on his inspired idea of inviting this influential man to our performance.

After this introduction I began teaching eurythmy. French and Russian students were the first to appear, adults as well as their children. In the lessons for the French students, I needed to live into the spirit of their language, which is so very different from German. Even the stepping of the French meters asked for a different kind of movement of the arms and posture of the body. For instance, the French language has a strong tendency toward the rising rhythm, toward iambic and anapaestic meter. In order to step the falling rhythm with my pupils, I had to turn to German and Latin texts.

Conveying the content of the language with the help of eurythmy posed great problems for me as well. I had received a few indications from Steiner for forming the French sounds, but since I had never taught in this language, I needed to start the eurythmy lessons afresh. Searching for texts for exercises for adults and for children from one lesson to the next was not an easy task. Sometimes I went into a lesson without having found the necessary texts. On the way to the Studio rue Huyghens, along the Boulevard Montparnasse, it often happened that an idea would come at the last moment: a missing sound or even a little poem that I composed and wrote down. So, for example, a little poem for children came to me that described how the colours come about through the working together of light and dark, but it was expressed in the same way as in Schiller's poem 'Riddle', which contains the fundamentals of Goethe's *Theory of Colours*. The poem began:

> *Nous sommes sept enfants mineurs,*
> *Trois frères et quatre soeurs;*
> *Le jour clair est notre père,*
> *La nuit est notre mère...*

(We are seven little children
Three brothers and four sisters
The clear day is our father
The night is our mother...)

The children were very pleased with it, as were their parents and the French members of the society.

At the end of March we were able to give a children's performance for members of our society and for invited families and guests. The children performed the opening exercises in their light green eurythmy dresses, fresh as spring leaves, their eyes radiant with joy and excitement. Simone Rihouët-Coroze sat next to the stage and accompanied the exercises with music that she had composed on a small Irish harp with green and gold decoration. A few poems were performed in the second part, among them my little colour poem which was done in the same way as Schiller's poem according to Steiner's indications in Dornach in 1917. At the front of the stage stood two taller figures: the 'mother' on the left (an older child) in a black dress and black veil, and the 'father' on the right (another older child) dressed completely in white. As with the performance of Schiller's poem, the mother did the dark vowels in the lines belonging to her, and the father did the light vowels in the lines belonging to him. In between them was the rainbow, with the children wearing coloured, cape-like collars that had been made for them. The four 'sisters' stood on the mother's side wearing violet, indigo, blue and green, and the three 'brothers' stood on the father's side wearing yellow, orange and red.

In the course of the poem they all moved around the stage (except for the two figures at the front) so that the seven different-coloured figures came into various relationships to each other. Then the seven children each did a small verse that was built on a specific vowel, conveying the essence of their particular colour. At the end there came a very funny poem with a tone eurythmy postlude, which was still at a primitive stage.

For the children, this performance was an important festive occasion, and it remains for me one of the most beautiful and radiant memories of my time in Paris. Unfortunately, our joy was marred by what happened next. Hardly had we finished when the audience's chairs were pushed aside to clear the floor. Rousing piano music started up and the audience began to turn and sway in a modern dance. The children were invited to join in, but they refused, pulling the curtain across the stage and hiding behind it. Despite their protests, some of the children were pulled from the stage by the adults, and pulled into the whirlpool on the dancefloor.

I relate this episode not in order to judge the people, but to contrast it especially with what the children had experienced just moments before. The adults were probably not aware of the up-building, healing spiritual forces that work on children when they do eurythmy. On many occasions, Steiner spoke of the effect this has on the whole soul nature soul of the child. He pointed to the fact that when performing eurythmy, children carry out movements that make it possible for divine spiritual beings to work on the growing human being. He said that you cannot teach anthroposophy directly to children, but that if they do eurythmy then through that they will be prepared for life in the right way. I was very sorry that on that afternoon the children were not taken home before that very different gathering had begun. Then, in the evening, they would have been able to take the festive, joyous mood with them into sleep.

Interest in eurythmy was increasing and we had to ask ourselves how we could develop the work further. The small studio on the rue Huyghens had room for a hundred people at most, with a stage so small it was difficult to move. Already in our first performances, we had great problems because of the small space, especially when it came to performing the group pieces. This was not the venue to present our art to a wider audience.

At Easter, I returned to Dornach for a short while. I told Marie Steiner about the difficulty of bringing proper performances to the Parisian public and representing eurythmy as a lively, buoyant spatial art of movement in such a small space. She listened with great interest, and when I returned to Paris I was tasked with looking for a larger venue for our anthroposophical work and especially for eurythmy. Soon afterwards, Simone Rihouët-Coroze found a space on the rue Campagne Première, in the artistic quarter of Montparnasse, that could be adapted for performances. It had a stage and an auditorium for more than two hundred people. We learned from the owner that the dancer Isadora Duncan, who was still living at the time, had also been interested in having her own theatre there. I wrote to Marie Steiner to inform her that a suitable space had been found and she telegraphed back that we should do everything necessary to acquire it. This exchange of letter and telegram between Marie Steiner and myself took place shortly before Whitsun. On Whitsunday, we celebrated with a eurythmy performance in which the students took part. It was the last one to take place on that small stage in the Studio rue Huyghens.

I returned to Dornach again at the end of June. Simone Rihouët-Coroze came soon afterwards to discuss the new space with Marie Steiner. She was accompanied by another Parisian eurythmist and the eurythmist's husband, who was an architect. The architect was given the task of carrying out the redecoration, and Marie Steiner generously covered the cost of the renovation and interior decorating herself. Simone Rihouët-Coroze and the couple soon returned to Paris and immediately began work to prepare the space for the winter season.

For my part, I was faced with all the legal difficulties of acquiring another entry permit to return to Paris. I turned to Alice Sauerwein, the General Secretary of the French national society, who had come to Dornach for Michaelmas. She wrote to me from Paris that it was out of the question that I would be allowed back. My files created an obstacle for my return, and she was unable to help me.

What was I to do?

By now the new space was completed and needed to be opened. It was high time to start with the performances and teaching. One night I had the thought that I should write a letter to the French minister. I did it immediately the next morning. A French artist studying in Dornach took on the task of giving this letter to an official he knew so that it should reach the minister. In this letter I told him confidentially about all the problems that I, a homeless Russian without the help and protection of a consul, had experienced. I told him my biography, about my previous activity in Paris and about the renovation of the new space. I also described the spiritual-scientific and artistic work at the Goetheanum and mentioned our artistic tours throughout Europe. I also told him that I worked with a group of Russians in my free time, in order to bring spiritual science to them. The *École Rudolf Steiner pour Science Spirituelle et Eurythmie* (Marie Steiner had given me permission to write this) would create the framework for further activity. With steadfast hope, I asked him for his help to investigate and remove all misunderstandings that obstructed my coming to Paris. I expressed my conviction that the truth was not hard to prove, and I ended the letter feeling confident that something so important for humanity would not be prevented from developing. A few days later a telephone call came from Paris, via the French consulate in Basel, granting me my entry permit from the minister. The continuation of the work was secured.

Eurythmy in other languages

While working with the vowels in the French language, it became apparent that the sun sound *AU*, which plays such an important role in the German language, does not appear in the French language at all. Instead the French have another diphthong which corresponds to the German, namely the frequently used *UA*, pronounced between *OA* and *UA*, and written *oi* in many important words, such as *moi, loi, roi, voix*. When I divided the vowels in the planetary circle according to the principle Rudolf Steiner had given for the seven vowels of the German language, it became apparent to me after placing the five basic vowels (*A, E, I, O, U*), and searching for the places for the diphthongs, that the French diphthong *UA* belongs in the same place as the German *AU*. I based this purely on the pronunciation of the diphthong, on the sound it makes: that is, half way between *A* (Venus) and *U* (Saturn). The only difference is that the German *AU* goes in the direction of the sun and the French *UA* in the direction of the moon, and whereas the German *AU* has something of a waning, descending character, the French *UA* has an ascending quality.

On the path of the moon the French vowel *OU* (*u*) is formed between *O* and *U* – for example, *nous, jour*. When doing orientation exercises and for poems built up according to this principle, the French word *soleil* (sun), with its emphasis on *ei*, would be in the realm of the moon, but moving in the direction of the sun – that is, from *O* (Jupiter) to *EI* (Moon). At the same place (Moon), one could do the French *je* (the word for I), which used to be pronounced closer to the German *ich*.

I Path of the Sun

II Path of the Moon

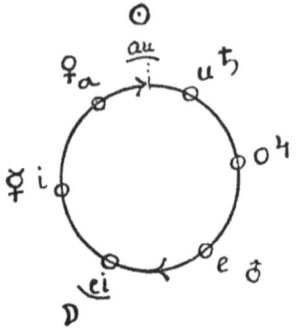
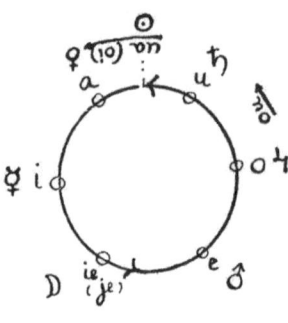

At the same time as I was giving a course in the French language, I also had to teach in Russian. That meant that I had to build up the lessons quite differently. The Russian language contains all the nuances of both rising and falling rhythms. It is rich in pure anapaestic poetry, which appears far less frequently in the German language. When stepping the meter in the Russian verses, it became apparent that Russian rhythms require less discipline and precision than is the case in German. I noticed this especially with the iambic, but also with the trochaic meter.

Steiner once pointed out that there are two basic underlying moods in Russian poetry that should be observed: asserting oneself and the opposite mood of complete devotion. The position of the fingers allows this contrast to come to expression. In the first mood all five fingers are held together, in the second the hand is opened with the first three fingers separate from the others.

Many years earlier, on October 31, 1905, Steiner had indicated that in the sixth cultural epoch, which he called the Russian-Slavonic epoch, the balance will be achieved between selfhood and selflessness: human beings will neither lose themselves in the outer world nor become shut off in themselves.[1] This balance, which the Russian language bears as a seed for the future, is especially revealed when the poems of Vladimir Solovyov are performed according to the indications given by Steiner.

The English language rests on another polarity: drawing toward oneself and energetically pushing away from oneself. This is expressed through corresponding gestures: the hands first directed strongly towards oneself and then sending them far from oneself, almost throwing them away from oneself. During a rehearsal in London, Steiner said that when performing poems in English, one must do larger gestures, to create the impression of expanding further out.

Concerning the special qualities of eurythmy when performed in the Russian language, Steiner said that the Russian and

German languages have a relationship to one another in that the speech sound with which a German word *begins* is in many instances the speech sound with which the corresponding Russian word *ends*, and vice versa. So for instance, the words *Gott* and *Bog* (God), or *oben* (up) and *nebesa* (heaven). There is also a certain relationship between *T* and *B*.

In my eurythmy notebook Steiner wrote the letters that show how the letter I is connected to J (or Y) in Russian. In the time since Peter the Great, when the upper class became strongly westernised, including the emigrants, many unfortunately lost the feeling for their own language, something Marie Steiner strongly condemned. Once when Rudolf Steiner was comparing languages to musical instruments, he said of the Russian language, 'At some point it will become a harp, but at present it is a zither.' I experienced something of this whenever Marie Steiner gave recitations in that language: her Russian already sounded like a harp. It all depends on the kind of consciousness with which the Russian meets the West.

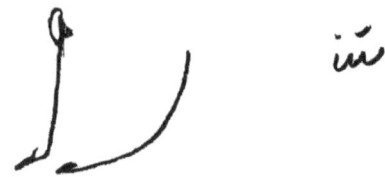

The content of Russian speech sounds, both vocalic and consonantal, differs greatly from German. It is even further away from the French. The diphthongs *AU* and *UA* (written *oi* in French) do not occur; one does indeed find a few words in Russian with the *AU* sound, but the emphasis is not on *A* but *U*, as for instance *naúka* (science) and *paúk* (spider). These appear very infrequently. In order to introduce my pupils to the sevenfold scale of the circle of vowels, I began bringing examples from three languages: French, Russian, and German. I did this in both French and Russian lessons. This awoke an interest in my pupils for the characteristics of the languages and for the different essential qualities of a folk. Later I also included Polish.

Starting in 1928 I began working with Germans who lived permanently in Paris or who were visiting for a period of time. It was always a great joy for me to give lessons in German. Although my command of it was far from perfect, it was much easier for me; I believe I was better at translating German texts into eurythmy as compared with French or even Russian. In this connection I would like to point out that Steiner spoke about the genius of the German language as containing a strong sculptural element.[2] Based on this, it is understandable that eurythmy came about in the German language, because eurythmy itself is moving sculpture and the sculptural can be formed most easily in the German language. Originally all languages had this moving plasticity.

In a lecture he gave on March 29, 1919, Steiner said:

> There is of course an enormous difference in the soul life, whether by the word Kopf something round, that is the form, is to be understood, as most noun formations in German are plastic imaginations, or whether, as in Latin languages, most noun formations originate in the presence of man, how he places himself into the world, not by perception but by placing himself into the world. Great mysteries lie hidden in language.[3]

I experienced this especially strongly for myself when I was teaching in three languages and searching for the meaning of the sounds in French and Russian.

Every language expresses a particular temperament and character. The French language, according to Steiner, was once a feeling or heart language, but it has since become more abstract. It is also true that the German language, in the course of its development, has moved much further away from being a 'living' speech than is the case with other western languages. In the lecture he gave in Stuttgart on December 29, 1919, Steiner spoke about the three metamorphic stages in the development of languages. At the first stage a language is adapted instinctively to the outer world, at the second it becomes soulful, and at the third it becomes spiritual, but in such a way that this inwardness produces an inner alienation from life. The German language, Steiner said, was at the third stage:

> The ascent to the third step that you can study especially in modern German ... is more a distancing from life, so that by means of its words such abstract heights can be reached as were reached, for instance, by Hegel, or also in certain cases, by Goethe and Schiller. That is very much dependent on this reaching-the-third-step. Here German becomes an example. The language-forming, the language-development, frees itself from attuning to the external world. It becomes an internal, independent process. Through this the human-individual soul element progresses, which, in a sense, develops independently of nature.[4]

How is it now with the Russian language? In the second lecture of the cycle *Speech and Drama*, Steiner speaks about the sign-like nature of European languages:

> The languages of Europe today – with the possible exception of Russian and a few languages less widely spoken, which have not as yet come quite so far away as the rest – the European languages generally are by this time very far removed from their origin, and they are spoken in such a way that the words and even the intonation of the sounds have become nothing more than an external sign for the experiences that originally gave rise to them.[5]

The re-enlivening of speech, to make the speech sound a revelation of the spirit, was the joint task of Rudolf and Marie Steiner.

In connection with Steiner's views about the development of language, I would like to draw attention to some further peculiarities of the sound qualities of the Russian language, without attempting to determine the level on which it stands because that would entail a comprehensive and detailed study which I cannot make. Nevertheless, I would like to present a few characteristic examples in order to call forth a picture of the sound element in the Russian language.

Let us take the eurythmy exercise, 'I think speech'.[6] For the final position and gesture, the eurythmist stands with their legs together and they arms held straight up in the air. This is the eurythmical expression of the vowel *U*. In German this position is accompanied by the words, '*Ich bin auf dem Wege zum Geiste*' ('I am on the way to the spirit'); in French by '*la voie vers l'Esprit*', and in Russian by '*Put' k Duchu.*' The threefold *U* that occurs here as done in eurythmy brings the human being exactly into the position given for the sixth and final sentence of the exercise.

Let us look at words like *uzkiy*, meaning narrow, and *umirayu*, meaning dying. The *U* sound expresses a narrowing, a stiffening, that which makes one cold, whereby one freezes. Now let us contrast this with the French word *étroit*, which also means narrow and is pronounced with the *UA* sound discussed above. Here we have, instead of a narrowing, an opening up due to the emphasis on the *A* sound at the end.

The vowel *U* is experienced as a going out of oneself and wanting to connect with the spirit:

> The feeling of *U* is that of being bound up with something, yet wishing to get away from it; following the movement you make and going somewhere else, leaving yourself and preparing your way. I run along my arms when I make the movement for *U* ... I stream away.

With both *O* and *U* there is:

> ... a distinct going-out of the soul from the body ...
> It really is a falling-asleep-while-still-awake when we utter *O* or *U*, or when we do *O* or *U* in eurythmy.[7]

Of further interest in this respect is the Russian word *budu*, or 'I will', the intention to carry out a future action. It is identical to the sound of the Indian word *Buddhi* or Life Spirit. And so when a person pronounces *budu*, they are already seeking the spiritual element of the future, even if they are not aware of it and resist hearing anything about it.

Speaking of the Russian language Steiner said that it is:

> ... a language which is merely suggestive, which only gives a faint indication of the inner nature of the word. It is a language which does not yet have its true being, but is following the tracks leading it towards this being, and everywhere points towards the future.[8]

In contrasting the French and Russian languages, Steiner said that with the Russian:

> ... you *follow on the tracks of the essence of the word* ... with the French there is *a tripping along in front of the essence of the word*.[9] (Italics in the original.)

Russian and French are therefore polar opposites.

Now I would like to draw attention to other properties of vowel qualities in the Russian language, such as, for instance, the role played by the vowels *I* and *O*. The sound *I* appears frequently, especially in its abbreviated form *Y*. So, for example, *I* often serves as the plural: *on* (he), *oni* (they); *knig* (book), *knigi* (books), and so on. In addition, *I* attached to the root of the verb makes the imperative: *idi* (go).

The short *Y* continuously accompanies the other vowels, sometimes coming before the vowel, as in *ya, ye, yi, yo, yu,* and sometimes coming before and after, as in *yey* (dative for *her*). The Russian *E* is mostly pronounced *yay*. All of this adds a strongly subjective note because the addition of *I* to the main vowel means the human being always keeps their own self in view. Thus their soul is in danger of losing itself in the purely individual-personal element and not experiencing the objective-spiritual element. If one is conscious of this danger, then one can battle with this tendency in the soul so that, in spite of the nuance given to experiences through the personal element, an objective attitude to impressions of the world is still possible.

A certain balance to this frequent appearance of *I* or *ye* is the many countless words in the Russian language that only contain the vowel *O*. No other language, as far as I know, has so many words with *O*. In this way the 'pure self-assertion' of *I* is counteracted by an understanding attitude that 'brings us into a more intimate relationship to what we perceive' through love for its being.[10]

There is a remarkable prevalence of *O* in words that pertain to the upper parts of the human being, for example: *golova* (head), *lob* (forehead), *brov^y* (eyebrows), *rot* (mouth), *podborodok* (chin). It is less prevalent in words for other parts of the body, for example: *pozvonok* (vertebra), *nogi* (feet). Then there are words with two or three *O*s: *mnogo* (a lot), *dovolno* (enough), *dorogoy* (expensive), *dobrovolno* (free will). Even with these few examples one can discern that the Russian language is an *O*-language *par excellence*. In many rural parts of Russia people still pronounce the *O* (at least it was so until recently), whereas in the big cities, especially among the educated classes, people pronounce most unstressed *O*s with an *A* sound: for example, *Maskva* instead of *Moskva* (Moscow), *galava* instead of *golova* (head).

When I asked Rudolf Steiner if we should follow the pronunciation of the educated classes or the language as it is written when performing poems in eurythmy, he said that in eurythmy one should do all *O*s, including the unstressed ones. He added that the pronunciation of *O* as *A* was a sign of decadence, a tendency found not only in Russian but in other languages as well. On the other hand, with the consonant *V*, especially at the end of a word, such as in the names *Petrov* and *Lvov* and so on, one should pronounce it not as it is written, but follow the common Russian usage where *V* is pronounced *F*: so *Petrof* (or, even better, *Petroff*) instead.

For the English language in eurythmy one should stick to the pronunciation of both vowels and consonants and never to how they are written down. The same applies to the French language (*eu* = E, *ou* = U, *oi* = UA, *il est* = IL E, and so on).

The German language is again rich in *E* words, especially words only containing the vowel *E*, possibly even richer than Russian words with *O*. According to Steiner the feeling inherent in *E* signifies:

> ... holding yourself upright while facing something ... we do not simply allow the world to approach us, but we offer some resistance ... We touch ourselves. We say, as we experience the *E*-sound, 'I too am here confronting the world.'[11]

In German there are a great many words, especially verbs, that only contain *E*: *estrebenswert* (worth striving for), *entgegenstellen* (oppose), *weltenwesen* (world being), *Erdenwerden* (earth becoming), *Menschenseele* (human soul).

That does not mean that the other vowels in the German language are irrelevant. The sun sound *AU* (or *I*, see p. 114) plays an even greater role than in probably any other language. Not only do we find the diphthong *AU* in such important words as *schauen* (watch), *bauen* (to build), and *vertrauen* (trust), but also in the prepositions *auf* (on), *aus* (out of), which are added before or after other roots where something of a sun quality plays through them, if I may put it like that. For example: *aufstehen* (stand or get up), *aufleben* (revive, become lively), *ausreifen* (mature), *hinauf* (up), and *hinaus* (out). This justifies seeing German as a language strongly imbued with sun impulses. For the other sun sound, *I*, see Christian Morgenstern's poem, '*Die Sonne will sich siebenmale spiegeln...*' ('The sun wishes to be mirrored seven times...').

Something I see as being particularly important is that in most words in which the quintessential German soul disposition comes to expression, especially the Goethean disposition as symbolised by *Faust*, the emphasised *E* also occurs next to the unstressed *E*: *streben* (strive), *werden* (become), *erkennen* (know) and so on. The German people always re-enliven themselves in the Faustian manner:

> However, we always know one thing: can it be
> we are already 'Germans'? That we cannot yet
> be. That we must eternally strive to become! The
> German knows that that which hovers in front of
> him as 'German' is an *ideal* which is connected to
> the deepest source of the spirit, that one *becomes* a
> German, always *becomes* but never is.

To that belongs the decision to strive *with* Goethe:

> Then the soul will be transported into those worlds
> that are here represented as what is meant by
> spiritual science.[12]

Russian also has *E*-words, though they are more seldom, but the *E* as already mentioned is pronounced *YE* or *YO*. There are a few pure *E*s. For instance *eto* (this), or *poet* (poet).

The French *E* has different nuances and appears frequently: *e* alone, *é* with acute accent, *è* with grave accent, *ê* with circumflex, and *ai* similar to the German *ä* (as in English 'hair'): *première, préféré, être, j'étais*. We tried to express all these nuances in eurythmy.

Another difference between the sounds of Russian and western European languages is the contrast between the pronunciation of hard and soft vowels and consonants. In the

Russian language the consonants at the beginning, middle or end of the word are pronounced hard or soft: soft before *I* and before the frequently recurring soft *E* (*ye, yo*), then also at the end of the word when a character known as the 'soft sign' – ь '(transliterated in English as *y*)' – stands after the last consonant of the word, or in the middle of the word. The word *vnov* (вновь), meaning 'again', has a hard *V* at the beginning and a soft *V* at the end. The hard sign at the end of a word (nowadays it is no longer used) makes the last sound hard: *nov*.

But the big difference in pronunciation is the sound *L* where the *L* is so hard that a non-Russian can hardly pronounce it. At the same time there are sound combinations that are possibly softer than in any other European language, such as in the word *lebed*^y, which means swan. This contrast between the pronunciation of hard and soft can be shown with another example: the vowel ы, which sounds especially hard. When I asked Rudolf Steiner how I should do this in eurythmy, he said '*ui, ui*' a few times and then led it over into the vowel ы. In this sound, the sounds *UI* are found in a melted state, it is not a diphthong. Due to the fact that I was working simultaneously with the Russian and German languages, I concluded that there are three steps in the pronunciation of sounds. Let us take three vowels:

Russian:	German:	Russian:
1. *Ty* (you)	2. *Tisch* (table)	3. *Tichiy* (quiet)

The German word *tisch* belongs in the middle between the very hard *ty* and the very soft *tichiy*.

| 1. hard: *ty* | 2. transition: *ti* | 3. soft: *tichiy* |

One finds the same three transitional steps from hard to soft pronunciation also after the consonants *B*, *D* and *R*:

Russian:	German:	Russian:
Byt^y (to be)	*Bitte* (please)	*Bitva* (battle)
Dym (smoke)	*Dick* (thick)	*Dikiy* (wild)
Rys^y (fox)	*Riss* (tear)	*Ris* (rice)

Rudolf Steiner indicated how this strong polarity can be expressed eurythmically if, when forming the hard consonants, the right arm and hand (and through that the whole right side of the body) are more strongly active than the left so that the overall movement is oriented towards the right; the right arm must also be kept close to the body. By contrast, with the soft consonants the left side predominates, especially the arm and hand, and the movements are more relaxed and further away from the body.

When observing and pondering the peculiarities of the sounds of the Russian language, one can say that the large number of soft consonants – designated in the western European languages as *mouillierte* – and the presence of the soft sign, especially at the end of a word, give the Russian language an overall soft sound. The hardness comes about only through the vowels *A, O, U*, especially *UI* (ы), and also through the hard sign found at the end and sometimes in the middle of the word, though rarely.

In the German language, all consonants at the end of the word, and nearly all in the middle, are spoken hard. An exception to this is in the softening of the consonant before the vowel *I*. All other German vowels, especially *E*, are hard sounds.

In a certain way one could say that hard and soft pronunciation in the Russian language holds a balance, with perhaps a slight predominance of the soft element, and that in the German language the predominance lies on the side of the hard element.

In addition to this polarity, there are also the contrasting directions of 'up' and 'down' in Russian texts in eurythmy. According to Rudolf Steiner's indication, when doing a poem by Vladimir Solovyov in eurythmy, the beginning of every line is in the lower or middle zone, then, in the second half of the line, we raise our arms to the level of the head or above it and perform the sounds, then we go back down again.

I have already mentioned the reversal of the sounds in the Russian and German languages (for example, *Bog/Gott* for God). In a conversation I had with Steiner during a rehearsal, he drew my attention to a peculiarity of the Russian language: the addition of the word *ya* (the pronoun *I*) to the names of animals, for example, *svinya*, the word for pig, with emphasis on the *A*. The word for snake, *smeya*, also has this *ya*. From Steiner's spiritual investigation we know that the snake appeared in earth evolution during the period when the spine was formed, when the nervous system became enclosed in the column of bone. This is the basis for selfhood. Previously there had only been spineless animals. The snake has therefore remained at the stage when the spine was being formed.[13] This *ya* is also in the word for monkey, *obezyana, O bez* (without) *ya* (I) *na*, or 'O without-I'. We know from anthroposophy that the ancestral animal of monkeys had an I, but then lost it. In the Russian language this loss is expressed even in the name.

Steiner said that in this context *ya* has a deep connection with Russia's special task, one that relates to the Parsifal-problem and the appearance of foolishness: Parsifal is 'the pure fool'.

This study, comparing sounds with the help of eurythmy, remained at an initial stage for the first few years. I had intended to continue the work with a linguist who was in Paris for a while, but unfortunately nothing came of it. In those days I experienced how working with eurythmy can help one regain a concrete connection to language, especially when one can do it simultaneously in a number of languages. through the possibility of doing gestures in a special way, deepening the sounds through the movement of the limbs, because one does not feel the soul, the spirit anymore in the sound directly.

One must not lose sight of the fact that in present-day languages, both the vowels and consonants are no longer immediate expressions of experiences as was the case in the distant past when human beings first started to speak. At that time, across the whole of the earth, a primal language was spoken that has since become lost, although according to Steiner a reflection of it can still be found even now in all languages:

> Every language contains certain sounds reminiscent of it; in fact, our modern languages are the relics of the primeval, universal language.[14]

Eurythmy in oriental languages

In previous years we had received indications from Steiner for the gestures of arms, hands, and fingers, and for the different zones, for forming the sounds for poems in oriental languages. As with western languages, the indications were different depending on the language. For example, in the ancient Egyptian language, gestures were more rigid, with the hands and fingers stretched and kept in and wrists immovable wrists; the thumb covered the palm, touching the little finger. For Chinese, fingers were still held together, but less strictly, everything was more relaxed and the wrist flexible. Movements and gestures were performed mainly in the area of the nose, ears, and larynx. For Japanese, the fingers were even more relaxed, able to form a more rounded gesture.

If you follow these indications, then the differentiated style of walking and overall carriage of the body and the head for each language come of their own accord. We performed oriental poems in German and French translations, and occasionally as free renderings. Unfortunately, we never managed to do the texts in the original languages. Steiner said that the attempts of modern artists to represent oriental dance by studying and imitating old works of art leads to quite other results than what can be achieved through eurythmy.

One eurythmist came to Steiner wanting to do a dialogue between Krishna and Arjuna from the *Bhagavad Gita* in eurythmy. Steiner said that to perform in the Indian style, one would need to develop a kind of belly-eurythmy. 'But we would rather spare ourselves that, wouldn't we?' he added.

If, with the help of anthroposophy, we concern ourselves with the ancient Indian culture, it becomes clear why Steiner spoke about belly-dancing. The first post-Atlantean culture, the ancient Indian epoch, stood under the sign of Cancer, which is related to the Moon, which has its house in this sign. The constellation of Cancer corresponds to the chest region in the human being, but the Moon corresponds to the sexual realm. This resulted, through the breathing process, in a sensitivity to everything that approached human beings as the elemental world on the one hand, and a worldview that emerged from out of the sexual sphere on the other. According to Steiner:

> At the time this was right, for a naïveté then existed which in later, corrupt ages was no longer there.[15]

Consonants in the sequence of human evolution (II)

Working through the two lecture cycles that Rudolf Steiner gave in 1924, *Eurythmy as Visible Speech* and *Speech and Drama*, I was prompted to work further with the sequence of consonants he had given in 1915.

BMDN / RL / G / CH F S H / T

I noticed that this sequence begins with four plosives, *B, M, D* and *N*, and ends with four fricatives, *CH, F, S* and *H*, leading over again to the plosive sound *T* or *TAO*: 'significantly streaming from above downwards' or 'it has struck'. One could say of *T* that it is a starting point like *B*, but on a higher level: *B* is 'the enveloping' and *T* is 'from above streaming downwards and touching'. The vibrating wave-like sounds *R* and *L* lie between the groupings of plosives and fricatives. The *G* has two pronunciations in German. In the word *gierig* (greedy), the first *G* is a plosive while the softer second *G* goes over towards *CH*, a fricative. An equivalent word in English would be 'gorgeous', where the first *G* is plosive and the second is fricative.

Steiner said that plosives have a self-assertive quality, the attitude of soul is one of egotism: the human being asserts themselves over the outer world and wants to retain their own human individuality. The fricatives on the other hand have a quality of self-sacrifice: the human being goes along with the outer world. As for the undulating wave-like sounds *R* and *L*, Steiner says:

> We need them when we wish to express neither merely the merging with the outer world, nor the mere strengthening of the self, but something which has movement actually inherent within it.[16]

Thus we have at the beginning of this sequence *B*, *M*, *D* and *N*, the one-sided, egoistic element; in the middle we have *R*, which is egoistic and 'does not yield up what it has created to the outer world, but retains it for itself and in itself', and *L*, the 'sound of reflection, but with devotion', which is already a transition towards the fricatives or breath sounds:

> In reality the breath sounds express sympathy with the outer world and the plosives sympathy with oneself. The breath sounds are non-egoistic; the plosives are egoistic.[17]

In many of his lectures, Steiner maintained that everything belonging to the development of humanity begins with egoistic affirmation – with asserting, with taking – and leads eventually to devotion and an altruistic release. But before a person can be empowered to make a healing sacrifice, they must first have developed inwardness – indicated by *R* and *L*.

In *Speech and Drama*, Steiner considers the same problem from another point of view: the connection to the four elements. He says that the plosives always strive toward the earth element, they correspond to the element of earth. The *L*, a wave-like sound, is connected with the fluid element, and *R*, a vibrating wave sound, corresponds to the element of air. The fricatives live in the element of fire or warmth.[18]

We can see form this that the life of the elements is also contained in this sequence of consonants: beginning with a hardening and a connection to the earthly, followed by an unfolding of the inner life that dissolves with the fire element into that which expands in heights and widths, the sequence rounding off and ending in *T*, streaming from above downwards in order to become earthly again. *TAO* represents the weight that creatively streams down, directed from heaven to the earth.[19]

Through the study of anthroposophy one will come to ever-deeper insights into this sequence of consonants, which Steiner said contained everything. Here I only wanted to draw your attention to what resulted from my work with these twelve sounds.

The World Clock

On January 3, 1918, I received a page from Rudolf Steiner's notebook on which he had written correspondences between the vowels and the planets: twelve different combinations (see p. 114, Vowels and the planets).

As these new indications went further than the ones we had received three years earlier, I asked him for some guidance. He spoke about the movement of the planets, how they entered into relationship with the constellations of the zodiac and how there were relationships between specific planets and certain constellations.

In January, 1918, Rudolf Steiner gave a series of lectures that later appeared under the title *Ancient Myths and the New Isis Mystery*. In the fourth lecture, held on January 8, this problem of the connection of the sounds with the planets and the relationship of planets to the zodiac was resolved, or at least an indication of the complete solution was given. Before I examine this problem more closely, I must refer to a few thoughts from these lectures.

In the two first lectures Steiner speaks about the nature of mythical thinking. He refers to the fact that an awareness of the connection between the human being as microcosm to the universe as macrocosm is the foundation for all mythical events. He speaks about the cosmic wisdom of the ancient Egyptians, the worldview of the third post-Atlantean cultural epoch, when the spiritual in nature was experienced directly through atavistic imaginations. Then Steiner moves on to the fifth post-Atlantean cultural epoch, the one we are currently in, and indicates that what was present in the Egyptian-Chaldean times, in the third post-Atlantean cultural epoch, must be repeated again in some form in our time. There must be a looking back towards the ancient time of imaginative consciousness, the Osiris time of ancient mythology:

> Human beings must find the way back again to the Imaginations ... we must find forms of experience that are common to the dead and the living.[20]

The path to these forms of experience is indicated in this lecture cycle.

In the fourth lecture, Steiner shows how precisely human beings in the fifth post-Atlantean epoch can find their way to the spiritual world, the way to their truest, highest human goal. They must place themselves in a new way into connection with the whole universe and the constellations of the universe. Just as we adjust ourselves to the clock that is regulated by the position of the sun, Steiner says that likewise we have:

...subconscious members of our human nature which take their direction from other constellations than those we go by when in physical life we set our clock by them.[21]

Steiner then proceeds, as an illustration, to place 'a piece of the World Clock' in front of us.

During the first five post-Atlantean cultural epochs, forces stream down from out of the universe that correspond to aspects of the human being. It has already been mentioned that Steiner said the ancient Indian culture stood under the influence of Cancer, and that this was connected to the chest in the human being (see section: Eurythmy in oriental languages). This sign is also related to the Moon, which has its home, its house, in Cancer. This constellation Cancer-Moon signifies a specific connection that the human being has to the natural world and their fellow human beings; it gives a special nuance to that epoch's worldview.

Steiner then goes on to show how successive cultural epochs stood under different constellations: the Persian epoch under Gemini-Mercury, the Egyptian-Chaldean epoch under Taurus-Venus, the Greco-Roman epoch under Aries-Mars, and our own epoch under Pisces-Jupiter.

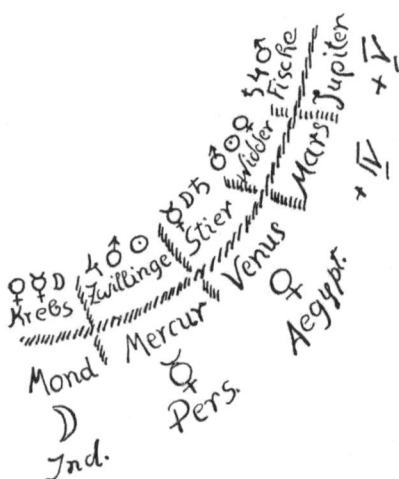

On this World Clock we see that every planet, known in earlier times as a Regent, has a specific group of planets in its sphere. Steiner said that those who understood the constellation of stars always knew that for the single divisions in the path of the sun, helping forces from specific planets streamed down. One called these helpers decans, and in every division there are three.

As regards the sources of present-day scientific knowledge about the constellations, and for guidance in finding the appropriate literature, I owe the following to Joachim Schultz. The division of the zodiac into 36 decans (or divisions of 10 degrees) has its origin in Egyptian culture and is reflected in the Egyptian calendar that existed already in 3000 BC. An Egyptian year had 12 months of 30 days, which were divided into 3 decans of 10 days each, so that 36 decans make a year. The assignment of the planets in a specific order to the 12 signs of the zodiac and to the 36 decans has been known since the end of antiquity and was taken over by astronomy in the Middle Ages.

This fivefoldness of the stars – the zodiac sign with its reigning planet and three decans – decide the inner mission or destiny of the age. There are twelve such five- membered constellations.

Since that time I have not ceased to busy myself with these connections, but many years passed before achieved results. I was certain that the two sequences of vowels, from Saturn *U* on the one side to Mercury *A*, and then again from Saturn *A* forwards to Mercury *U*, must stand in connection with the World Clock mentioned in that lecture.

Saturn – *U*   Saturn – *A*
Jupiter – *O*   Jupiter – *E*
Mars – *I*   Mars – *I*
Venus – *E*   Venus – *O*
Mercury – *A*   Mercury – *U*
Moon – *I-EI*
Sun – *I-AU*

The portion of the World Clock that Steiner drew invites completion with the further constellations: Saturn in Aquarius, Saturn in Capricorn, Jupiter in Sagittarius, Mars in Scorpio, Venus in Libra, Mercury in Virgo, and Sun in Leo. Then one has the complete World Clock.

Onto this completed World Clock, I then added the planets Steiner had given me in his list, beginning with Saturn *U* in Aquarius and (following the eurythmical path of the sun) passing through Jupiter *O* in Pisces, Mars *I* in Aries, Venus *E* in Taurus to Mercury *A* in Gemini and Moon *EI* in Cancer.

After that came the second combination, starting from Saturn *A* in Capricorn and proceeding right to Jupiter *E* in Sagittarius, Mars *I* in Scorpio, Venus *O* in Libra, Mercury *U* in Virgo. Then, once, the Sun *AU* in Leo and the Moon *EI* in Cancer.

The houses and decans of the zodiac

The decans begin with Aries-Mars and then, going down, follow the planetary spheres: Sun, Venus, Mercury, Moon, and so on, rhythmically repeating through the whole zodiac. At Pisces it does not end, but ends again with Mars, so that Mars appears twice in succession.

In the following drawing the heavens are depicted in two halves, as was done in ancient times. Every planet has two houses in the zodiac, a 'day house' and a 'night house'. The bottom half of the circle begins on the left with Cancer and proceeds through Gemini, Taurus, Aries and Pisces to Aquarius, and embraces the night houses of Moon, Mercury, Venus, Mars, Jupiter and Saturn. The top half begins with Leo and proceeds through Virgo, Libra, Scorpio and Sagittarius to Capricorn, and embraces the day houses of Sun, Mercury, Venus, Mars, Jupiter and Saturn. Sun and Moon are one-sided rulers of the day and night, so each needs only one house: Leo belongs to the Sun, Cancer to the Moon. On the other hand,

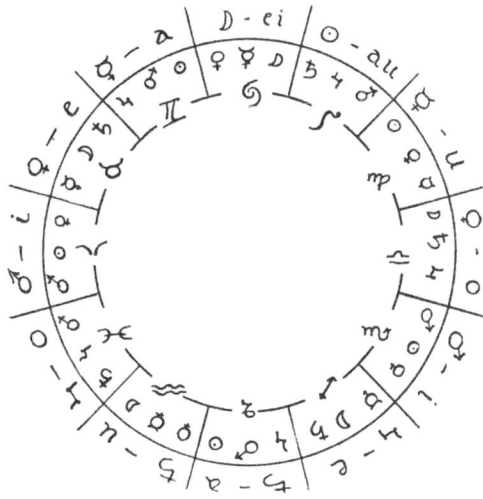

each actual planet has two houses. The Moon is the leader of the night houses, the Sun the leader of the day houses.

By engaging myself with these configurations, I was able to understand why Mars is the only one of the planets to carry the same sound, *I*. Mars in Aries and Mars in Scorpio (its day and night houses) carry exactly the same decans next to them, namely Mars, Sun, Venus. With all other planets the decans change (see above diagram).

There are aspects of this World Clock that are still not quite comprehensible, but I hope that with further work one thing after another will be clarified. The fact that Rudolf Steiner's remarks about the houses and decans of the zodiac came at the same time as the conversation during which I received the page from Steiner's notebook referred to above, makes me think that Steiner had just these configurations in mind.

During the first eurythmy course in Dornach in 1915, Steiner gave only the first five of the twelve connections that I later received from him in 1918, namely for the dance of the planets that we were practising at the time, so Saturn *U*, Jupiter *O*, Mars *I*, Venus *E*, Mercury *A*. Then, in 1924, during the Speech Eurythmy Course, we received another set of connections of vowels and planets: Saturn *U*, Jupiter *O*, Mars *E*, Mercury *I*, Venus *A*.

I am of the opinion that, for the time being, the connections Steiner gave in 1918 should remain insofar as they relate to the specific aspects of the World Clock I have mentioned here. Nor do I feel it is right to replace what was given for the dances of the planets (for which Steiner also gave corresponding colours) with new connections. My contribution to the question concerning the connection of the planets to the signs of the zodiac is to be regarded as one indication regarding this important problem and as a stimulation for further work.

Eurythmy in Rudolf Steiner's Mystery Dramas

As has been mentioned, Rudolf Steiner inaugurated a new art of spiritually appropriate movement with the first performance of the Mystery Drama *The Guardian of the Threshold* in Munich in August, 1912. In the sixth scene of the drama, two separate groups of thought-beings appear in a dance-like manner, one from Lucifer's side and the other from Ahriman's. In 1913, the use of the new art of eurythmy came a step further with the sylphs and gnomes in the performance of *The Soul's*

Awakening. Later, in Dornach, we received new forms and indications for both dances for eurythmy from Rudolf Steiner and soon afterwards the 'voice' and the soul forces who appear before and after the dance of the thought beings (in *The Guardian of the Threshold*, scene six). Also, in the second scene of the same drama, the soul forces and the voice of conscience were presented, with forms for eurythmy by Rudolf Steiner. I performed in scene seven of *The Portal of Initiation*. The fairy tales from the Mystery Dramas were also performed with forms and indications by Rudolf Steiner: 'The Fairy Tale of Love and Hate' from *The Portal of Initiation*; 'The Rock Spring Wonder' and the story about the tree and the axe from *The Soul's Probation*; and 'The Fairy Tale about Fantasy' in *The Guardian of the Threshold*.

After the opening of the Goetheanum, scenes were also performed from *The Soul's Awakening*: in the second scene, the appearance of the soul forces, which follows the sylphs and gnomes; Johannes's youth with Lucifer and Theodora, then the other Philia. Apart from Johannes and Theodora, who recited their parts without eurythmy, all others performed eurythmy with forms and indications by Rudolf Steiner. Marie Steiner recited the texts for the eurythmists. During the dance of the sylphs and gnomes, Johannes and a second figure in matching eurythmy garments accompanied the dance of the beings in the middle of the stage by creating the same forms with their arms as the beings created in space.

The fourth scene of the drama *The Soul's Awakening* was also performed. Johannes recited without eurythmy, the Double, the Guardian of the Threshold, and Ahriman were all performed in eurythmy, then Benedictus and Maria appeared, reciting without eurythmy. The Guardian of the Threshold had a crimson garment and a crimson Tao sign placed on the flowing hair of the performer.

The eurythmy costume for the part of Lucifer was made according to Steiner's indications. It consisted of a red undergarment with folds, and over this, instead of a veil, there was a cloud-like winged-larynx-ear structure. This top garment consisted of a wave-like creation: bigger waves for the wings going over into smaller waves where the ears, the larynx, and the forehead would be. Lucifer was also presented this way in the cupola painting as well as in the sculptural group by Steiner. Ahriman had a yellow garment, like the Ahriman performer in the Mystery Dramas, and a very tall head-piece, also in yellow.

In the introduction he gave before this performance, Steiner explained how the spiritual forces that play into the human soul throughout the course of an individual's biography, can best be grasped on stage with the help of the visible speech of eurythmy. On another occasion, in introductory words to scenes from *The Soul's Awakening*, Steiner pointed out that here the real self-knowledge of Johannes Thomasius is presented as his own being in image form. Johannes experiences his present being in image as his double, and this image of his youth, the 'spirit of Johannes's youth', as a second double. Both are objective figures, not abstract symbols or allegories. The Guardian of the Threshold, Lucifer and Ahriman are also not symbols but spiritual realities.

The Future of Eurythmy

On the night of September 28, 1939 I completed the first manuscript of my memoir. A huge fire raged across Europe. Nations were shedding their blood in mutual acts of destruction, and with the help of modern technology they were, with lightning speed, tearing down what had taken hundreds of years to build up. Hundreds of thousands of people were torn away from their work, were wounded, or killed. And not even a month had passed since the war broke out! In a few days, the Carpenter's Shop with adjoining rooms would once again be a home for anthroposophical work.

That was the last night that I would be able to spend in Rudolf and Marie Steiner's studio. I had been permitted to live there for a few weeks while I wrote my memoir, surrounded by the eternal spiritual realities of the years of activity of these two individuals in Dornach. I had only been able to describe the development of eurythmy in a faltering fashion; it did not lie in my powers to describe in more all-encompassing way this art of movement received from the spirit, nor to describe the sacrificial deed of Rudolf and Marie Steiner in other areas during those years when humanity was raised to spiritual heights.

Every time I am asked, or I ask myself, what is required for the right development of eurythmy and for keeping the art of eurythmy alive, Goethe's words from *Faust* come to mind:

> The things that we inherit come alone
> To true possession by the spirit's toil.[1]

We have been given this invaluable treasure, eurythmy. We must earn it in order to own it and, in the truest sense, be allowed to call ourselves 'eurythmists'.

I have mentioned how Rudolf Steiner was fond of saying, 'Test yourself, student, practise with great diligence!' and that we should make this our motto for everything. He was very strict in this sense. He advised eurythmists to practise the given movements over and over again, and rejected gestures whenever he felt the deeper experience of the soul-spiritual substance was lacking in the individual sounds. He called this 'signalling' instead of 'doing eurythmy'.

Concerning the law of repetition he said:

> Life is constant repetition. If the spiritual realm is to become truly alive ... we must imitate in our souls what the laws of life have formed in the physical world, which for all its ossified nature has a spiritual origin ... The saving grace – if I may use these emotive words – of humanity's spiritual development will be that people do not settle into relating to spiritual ideas in the way that this tends to happen today, an attitude that can be characterised by statements such as, 'Oh, I know that already, I have heard it all before,' but instead regard these ideas as being like life itself, which is always associated with repetition, with ... a recurrence of the same phenomenon at the same place.[2]

This repetition is the magical power that ultimately transforms the etheric body into Life Spirit.

Steiner had already mentioned that often when two beings or two individuals say the same words, something different or even at times entirely contradictory is said. What is important is 'the whole human-spiritual' context, who is speaking not just what is being said.[3] It is also thus with eurythmic speech movements. Outwardly, two eurythmists might do exactly what they have been asked to do and it looks similar, and yet it may well have a completely different effect on the onlooker (and also on the eurythmists). A person with clairvoyance and a being of the spiritual world will also perceive something quite different: the eurythmy gestures and movements appear to them devoid of soul and spirit. If the eurythmist fails to strive toward becoming a new human being (or better yet, becoming a *true* human being) by continuously testing and developing themselves, their gestures are nothing more than signals.

Developing in the direction of becoming a true human being presupposes a striving toward inwardness, toward a deepening of the inner life. In speech, the vowels correspond to this quality of soul or soulfulness: what lives inwardly in human beings is expressed through the vowels, we reveal ourselves in the vowels. In order to come closer to this feeling quality of the vowels, besides the various exercises eurythmists practise, I think there should also be a meditative experience of the vowels in the most significant words. We can see what is meant in the example of the vowel O. In the characterisation of the vowel O as 'lovingly embracing', Rudolf Steiner wrote *Bewunderung* – admiration, appreciation. The human being goes a little out of themselves while at the same time enclosing something. They identify themselves with that which they enclose in an inner attitude full of intimate understanding.[4] This belongs to the essence of sacrifice. I find it deeply significant and worthy of wonder that this emphasised O, through the spirit of the German language, has been placed in this word *Opfern* meaning sacrifice.

When we experience the O intensively and form it correctly in eurythmy, Steiner says that we become weak. I became aware that through the flowing out of the soul into the space enclosed by the gesture, the soul partially withdraws from the body. This is experienced as becoming weaker. Allowing all this to stream through the soul and placing it into the O sound leads to a further step on the path of development in eurythmy.

As I watch eurythmy performances nowadays, I notice again and again that most of the eurythmists do *Ah-O* instead of *O*, exactly as in 1924. During lectures on speech eurythmy, Rudolf Steiner spoke to a eurythmist who was demonstrating the *O* and drew her attention to it three times, made three attempts and said, 'That is not an *O*, but an *Ah-O*.' This makes me ponder, especially when I remember how once during a rehearsal of a verse from the Calendar of the Soul, Steiner was dissatisfied and wanted to withdraw the verse from the program Marie Steiner asked whether, after further diligent practice, it might be more acceptable, to which Rudolf Steiner answered, 'Yes, but it will only be good enough after a few incarnations!' Those involved with this were among the best eurythmists at the time.

I have mentioned that Rudolf Steiner said that eurythmy had to enter into human evolution out of necessity in the present time, but that this is no cause for pride. He brought eurythmy in connection with the lofty human member of Life Spirit and said, 'But of course at the moment this is something that will only reach some degree of perfection in the very distant future'[5] – only after a few incarnations!

But the development of the human being also requires nurturing an interest in material phenomena. Next to inwardness and the cultivation of the soul qualities – which, in speech, corresponds to the vowel element, to movement, feeling and emotion, not to activity – the human being must turn their gaze to the surroundings. If we only look into the inner life, we are unable to get away from our own personality. We can only come to our I by turning our gaze toward the human form as a whole; at present this is the only place where we can find an expression of our I in the outer world. As the plants and crystals are an expression of their being, so also the human form corresponds to the being of humanity and to the I that holds this being together.

During my activity in Paris we had monthly public performances on the stage of the École Rudolf Steiner, 6 rue Campagne Première. With the beginning of our anthroposophical work in this school, fierce attacks started against the person and work of Rudolf Steiner from certain Russian immigrants living in Paris. For example, in lectures held by the enemies of anthroposophy it would be said that Steiner had claimed he was the reincarnation of John the Baptist and that he had built a temple in Switzerland with the name Johannesbau for just this reason. Thereupon we decided to organise a public conference with the theme 'The Personality of Rudolf Steiner'. Two days before this conference began, our Russian friends pasted almost the whole town with big posters that announced six lectures and a eurythmy performance with Russian poetry and musical compositions at the end. The interest in anthroposophy grew from day to day. The eurythmy performance was very well attended and well received. Articles and reviews appeared in the newspapers. Many showed a familiar and characteristic lack of understanding, but to our great joy we read one that was full of sincere sympathy for this noble, unassuming art. The eurythmy performance in particular was noted by the writer who was not an anthroposophist:

> In the whole performance, in the choice of the musical as well as the poetic pieces, in the way of costuming, in the fact that the names of the artists were not mentioned ... in all this lies a youthful seriousness and innocence. I heard someone in the audience say, 'Eurythmy gives women back their original Idea, that which lived in the divine intention as the "woman" archetype.'

Mention is made here only of 'woman' because in that performance no men took part on the stage. I made a written report of this, describing the negative campaign against Rudolf Steiner that had proceeded our counter-attack. Marie Steiner thought it important that the report be printed in *Das Goetheanum* so that anthroposophists would learn of the energetic battle being fought against the enemies of our movement in Paris and the important part eurythmy played in the École Rudolf Steiner. Marie Steiner said to me, 'Such an article about eurythmy in Paris hits the nail on the head with its profound assessment of the matter as it has never before been said, which has never been written by a critic!' Marie Steiner was deeply satisfied. Despite this, however, my report never appeared in *Das Goetheanum*.

What joy it is, how hopeful and encouraging, to see the remarkable thoughts and experiences eurythmy, as imperfect as it may be, can generate in audiences today and the strong effect it can have. Rudolf Steiner says that true art has a stronger effect on people than moral education because what is eternal and immortal shines through it.

> Art is indeed ultimately the child of the gods which saves humanity from descending into mendacity.[6]

Thus the ideal or archetype resounds in art. When Steiner says that the human being does not fulfil their archetype, the earnest question then arises: to what extent is our outer form, or *Gestalt*, an illusion, and where is our falling away from the divine archetype especially strong?

For those who develop their powers of observation and a more refined and delicate sense of feeling, who do not give themselves over entirely to a wholly subjective, self-satisfied, sensuous existence, they experience that the human countenance is not as it ought to be.

> We learn to see how the human countenance and all that belongs to it – indeed the whole of the upper part of the human being – has undergone change in the course of time through the working of pride in the human soul – pride and haughtiness and presumption.[7]

Rudolf Steiner once said to me that it makes no difference whether a eurythmist is pretty or not; a pretty or good-looking eurythmist will look especially unsightly if their movements are superficial and performed without soul. In many instances it would be better if the eurythmist's expression is not enlivened or ennobled through the deepened experience of eurythmy, for their face to be covered by a veil or a mask or even by makeup. Steiner, who sometimes did the makeup himself, did it quite differently from the way ladies apply it in the outer world when they wish to appear beautiful and well presented. Some of the eurythmists who Steiner made up, and who still clung to their vanity, quickly redid their makeup, unobserved, before going on stage.

The lower half of the human organism should also have a different form. For the human being to come again to this original form, something else besides pride must be overcome: desire. Originally the human being was constituted differently, and the esoteric student said in turning away from this earthly form:

> You are false ... It is earth life that has made you as you are; the form in which we see you now refers us back to another and altogether different form.[8]

So the human form has been changed from the archetype, in the upper realm through pride and arrogance, and in the lower realm through desire. It is good if those practising eurythmy concern themselves with this problem.

In order to gain greater certainty about this inner experience, Steiner shows that the human form is made up of twelve members to which specific terms have been allotted. These terms are the names of the signs of the zodiac. The human form is divided into twelve parts that are, so to speak, the building blocks of the temple of the Divine. In connection with their *Gestalt* human beings are a temple that contains what is hidden of the spiritual world. The unity of the human form is therefore an illusion.

For the esoteric seeker it is safer to start with the *Gestalt* of the human being, because it is least influenced by the luciferic and ahrimanic forces, although they have won influence here as well.

In 1917 Rudolf Steiner gave us a diagram of the consonants in the zodiac, noting for every zodiac sign the corresponding consonant (see p. 116). In 1924 he added further indications.

Present in the consonants is an after-image of outward forms or external happenings; sculpturally, they endeavour to recreate the outer form of things. The forces of the consciousness soul develop, to begin with, through the observation and study of the outer world, of outwardly sense-perceptible things and events. If this is to lead to the forming of the living, essential being of the consonants in eurythmy, it must not produce merely an outward imitation of forms or events, which is the materialistic way of doing things today. The speech sounds are beings of a higher world whose inner development is mirrored in speech itself. Steiner said:

> In the same way as we observe the progression in
> the plant world from the greening leaf in spring
> and the burgeoning blossom, to the developing of
> the fruit and again to the decay, so the being from
> the hierarchy of the angels observes the progression
> of the speech sounds in the realm....of speech.[9]

Eurythmists should develop that organ, one that Goethe possessed to such a high degree, by which one can perceive and feel the spirit behind the appearances in the world of the senses. This is the spirit that speaks out of all of nature. To sculpturally recreate this sensory-supersensory reality is the activity of the consonants in eurythmy. This connection with the consonants in eurythmy and the spirit that speaks to us in nature, led Steiner to comment about the possibility of a eurythmist becoming a natural scientist in the next incarnation.

Concerning the arms and hands, Steiner:

> For the organs we call arms and hands would, if we studied them seriously, reveal in a high degree the sublime significance of the nature of the human being. If we wanted to speak of *art* in nature – and the whole of what humanity rightly regards as the Temple of God is wonderfully imbued with nature's art – we could find no better expression of it than in the marvellous construction of the hands and arms ... If we observe all that human beings have had to do in the course of evolution with their hands, we find them to be the most precious possessions. When it is a matter of bringing to outward expression what the mind and spirit are able to achieve, then the hands show their value.[10]

The means of expression in the art of eurythmy is the whole human being, but very especially the human hands. These words should awaken an exceptional feeling of responsibility in us!

A tremendous perspective that touches us in our deepest being is revealed when reading Steiner's words in his lectures about the Luke Gospel:

> We shall let our whole being be permeated by the Christ-principle and our hands will bring to expression what is living in our souls as a faithful picture of that principle. Our hands were not created by ourselves but by the Father-principle, and the Christ-principle will stream through them. As human beings pass through incarnation after incarnation, the spiritual power flowing from the Mystery of Golgotha will stream into what they achieve in their bodies – which are the creations of the Father-principle – so that the outer world will eventually be imbued with the Christ-principle.[11]

There is an especially interesting consonant that I would like to use to demonstrate what I mean when I speak of the re-creation of the essential in outer appearances and events. It is the speech sound *L*.

In the course on speech eurythmy in 1924, Steiner said:

> *L* is a very remarkable sound ... You become aware of a creative, form-giving element when you pronounce an *l* ... There is something creative, something form-giving in this sound.[12]

And later in the course:

> *L* was looked upon in the Mysteries as a sound possessing special magical qualities, for when you give form to something it follows that you have power over it.[13]

Now, what outer event corresponds to the sound *L*? It corresponds to the development of the plant from root to blossom, and so on. Steiner was dissatisfied with the way the eurythmists did this sound. Once he demonstrated the *L*. He lifted up the arms and hands with the fingers almost held together – about to the level of the eyes – and opened the fingers suddenly, abruptly, expanding the hands, the arms. Immediately afterwards he let the arms and hands fall slowly and said, 'Nature makes jumps.' And a jump in the process of growth from leaf to blossom – that is what he wanted to see in the eurythmy gesture for *L*. One cannot perceive physically this abruptness in the unfolding of the plant blossom and the beginning of wilting that immediately follows, but etherically it happens.

Concerning the sensible-supersensible being and becoming of the other consonants, I cannot go into that here unfortunately. For the sound *M* it would be especially interesting, with all the various ways of movement expressing that sound allows:

movement of the legs, knees, arms and elbows, and the movement in space, forwards and backwards. It is similar to swimming, which can also be done in various ways.

About *M* Rudolf Steiner says:

> *M* signifies the understanding of something, the capacity for intelligently entering into something ... in the *M* of the sacred Indian syllable *AUM*, there is expressed a marvellous understanding of the universe. *M* may be said to signify laying hold of something – first the feeling of laying hold of something, then penetrating into it and lastly understanding it. The position should be held for a moment, so that this intelligent comprehension, coming about as a matter of course, is shown at the end in the gesture. The arms should be held slightly in front of the body. It would indeed be wonderful if this movement could also be taught to elephants. An elephant could make a wonderful *M* by stretching its trunk out and then turning it under. You couldn't get a more perfect example of an *M*. An *M* carried out in this way would really be the best possible *M* imaginable. I mention all these things as they may help you to experience the sounds.[14]

An elephant could also do an *E* better than a human being:

> The experience of *E* has already gone through something. Something has happened, and the effects of this happening we experience in the gesture. You can only experience the movement for *E* when something has happened, if you feel something. You feel this something when one part of the human organism is brought into direct contact with another part in a gesture. Now, this

cannot be done in so many ways. Man is differently built, for example, from the elephant and is consequently not able to make his nose so flexible that with its tip he can touch his cheek. Were he able to do this, it would be a most excellent example of an *E*-gesture.[15]

In this humorous way Rudolf Steiner indicates our limitations, our incapacity to form the sounds in beautiful and varied ways. All of this would be a healthy remedy for those who take themselves too seriously and who feel superior in every way to other earthly beings.

Once Rudolf Steiner said that the horse was so organised as to make it impossible to do eurythmy. If it tried, it would become mad. The kitten, on the other hand, is so constituted that if intelligence were added, it would be able to do eurythmy very nicely. And the little monkey would be quite delightful!

It could not be more clearly stated that in the expression of our sounds we eurythmists were still very limited, and much else that we did was imperfect too. This should make us humble. Not only are we inhibited because our physical body is so hardened, our organism ossified and rather inflexible, but our etheric bodies are hard and inflexible as well. Rudolf Steiner said:

> Because Ahriman's presence in the world caused the human etheric body to become so hardened that we are unable to develop eurythmy as a natural ability, we must try to wrest this eurythmy from Ahriman. The human being would move in a eurythmy-like way if not for the fact that Ahriman has hardened the human etheric body to such an extent that the element of eurythmy cannot find its way to expression.[16]

What is important for me here is to indicate how we must learn to make our own what has been given to us as eurythmy.

A great deal is involved if we want to go from merely making signals to doing eurythmy properly. I have tried, at least in connection to speech eurythmy, to indicate what pertains to the perfecting of the art of eurythmy: what I think and feel, and how I imagine eurythmy's further development. In support of this, the many quotations from Steiner have appeared necessary to me. In my opinion it is most important that we take to heart all that Rudolf Steiner said in countless lectures, introductions and personal conversations – warning, cautioning, awakening, and showing the way for our souls.

In eurythmy, the whole human being is the instrument of the art. Outer skilfulness, purely manual dexterity, is not enough. The inner attitude with which we fill ourselves – the moral substance, the serious feeling of responsibility – is indispensable, just as it is for all the other arts.

There are many dangers on the path of the artist. For example after the first stage of development has been achieved, the danger is that we might lose our original freshness and enthusiasm, we no longer engage with challenges with the same intensity and constant wrestling. To receive praise and recognition from critics instead of mockery and derision, to be celebrated instead of discredited: these are strong temptations for the eurythmist of today.

Rudolf Steiner once said that if we received newspaper articles praising us, then we should ask ourselves whether we had perhaps made compromises in our work for the sake of popularity and favourable notices.

The following words by Steiner can only strengthen the soul of the eurythmist, and at the same time be a guiding star for their further path:

> Round about us, in the environment of soul and
> spirit which we shall absorb at a later stage, the Life
> Spirit is also present. Therefore one day the Life
> Spirit may be come to be lowered into the Spirit
> Self. But of course at the moment this is something

> that will only reach some degree of perfection in the very distant future, for when we try to lower the Life Spirit into the Spirit Self, we will have to be living in entirely in an element which as yet is absolutely strange to us. So what we can say in this domain is like the babbling of an infant before it has learnt to speak properly. One can foresee for the far distant future that there will be an art of great perfection that will stand out beyond poetry, as poetry stands out beyond music, music beyond painting, painting beyond sculpture, and sculpture beyond architecture – this being of course not a question of superiority but of arrangement. You will have guessed that I am referring to something of which we know only the most elementary beginnings today: ... the art of eurythmy.[17]

Taking to heart Rudolf Steiner's advice we must make the effort not just to read, but also to work through what is being offered, so that we progress from an outer receiving to an inner experience. This inner work is essential for real progress to take place.

When will the Life Spirit will be sunk into the Spirit Self?

We know that our I, the fourth member of the human being, will progress to the stage of full human development during the present incarnation of our earth planet. The I is the actual treasure of the earth, it is the mission of the earth to develop the I. The fifth member of the human being, the Spirit Self, will go through its development during the earth's next incarnation, Jupiter, and will emerge from the transformed astral body. The sixth member, the Life Spirit, will undergo its development on the incarnation following Jupiter, that of Venus, and emerge from the transformed etheric body. Now comes the big question: how are we to think about this sinking of the Life Spirit into the Spirit Self, that will take place in only the far distant future? How is this connected to eurythmy?

Let us make clear what has been said in the last paragraphs with the following diagram that Steiner gave in his lecture series *Art As Seen in the Light of Mystery Wisdom*:[18]

Physical Body	
	Architecture
Etheric Body	
	Sculpture
Astral Body	
	Painting
I	
	Music
Spirit Self	
	Poetry
Life Spirit	
	Eurythmy

Over the course of earth evolution the I, as the centre of the human being, gradually works on the astral body to transform it by degrees into Spirit Self. Steiner describes this process:

> The I transforms the astral body slowly and gradually into sentient soul, rational soul and spiritual soul. The I continues its work and it is only when it has taken the astral body to spiritual soul level that it is able to purify it so that Spirit Self may arise in it ... It is inseparable bound up with the spiritual soul, rather like a sword in its sheath ... Spirit Self is also Holy Spirit, in Christian terms the leading spirit on the astral plane ... The spiritual soul is the principle in which the Spirit Self has developed and is therefore called 'the mother of Christ' or in occult schools 'the virgin Sophia'.[19]

Steiner said that the astral body of every human being whose I has already worked on it, is divided into two parts:

the astral body as it was given to the human being and a part that has been worked over by their I. This transformed part, which increases in size the more the human being develops, is what is called Spirit Self. Esoteric Christianity identifies this part as the Holy Spirit, the 'pure, chaste, wise Virgin Sophia', and the Christian esotericist 'makes their astral body into the Virgin Sophia and is illuminated from above – if you wish, you may call it overshadowed – by the Holy Spirit, by the Cosmic, Universal Ego.'[20]

Similarly, the I works on the etheric body and transforms it into Life Spirit. In Christian esotericism this is also called the Word or the Son: Christ is the eternal part of the Life Spirit. This higher member is present in most human beings in seed form. The Spirit Self, the mother of the redeemer, the 'pure, chaste, wise Virgin Sophia', must first mature toward an understanding of the Christ impulse:

> Recalling again the five periods of civilisation – Indian, Persian, Egyptian, Graeco-Roman and European – we see that the basis for the Christ power that will bear fruit for the whole of humanity was established during the third period. The foundation then laid within human evolution will only emerge into life in the sixth period. Then the Spirit Self, which has evolved from the spiritual soul, will connect with the Life Spirit. From the third to the fourth period the Christ power shone out prophetically. In the sixth period, the great marriage of humanity will be celebrated as the Spirit Self unites with the Life Spirit.[21]

Rudolf Steiner said further that humanity would be united into one great brotherhood, which one finds prefigured in the description of the marriage at Cana in the second chapter of John's gospel:

Three periods have to pass from the third period before this will come to pass – the third, fourth and fifth. In esoteric teaching a period is called a day, which is why Chapter 2 begins with the words 'on the third day a wedding took place at Cana in Galilee.' The words indicate that the story of the wedding which follows refers to something that will happen in the future. The mother of Jesus, the spiritual soul, was present at the wedding. The Christ said to her, 'This is between me and you, woman, my hour has still not come.' This clearly shows that reference is made to something at the wedding in Cana that is due to happen only in the future.[22]

The future development of the Spirit Self will be prefigured in the sixth cultural epoch that will follow our current epoch. But the human being will not be able to develop it out of their own forces, they will not yet be able to call this Spirit Self their own. Instead they will experience how, after their I has undergone a certain development, a kind of angel being will illuminate this Spirit Self. Through the grace of higher beings it will become their guide. And it will be the same with Life Spirit in the seventh cultural epoch. The human being will speak about their Spirit Self and Life Spirit as of a higher nature that stands above them and to which they look up. They will prophetically anticipate what they will only make fully their own, what will only come to full development, on the Jupiter and Venus incarnations of our earth.[23]

In his introductory remarks to eurythmy performances given in July 1923, Rudolf Steiner shared important results of his spiritual research in connection with this prefiguring of the future Jupiter and Venus developments. When the human being accompanies his speech with gesture in order to give his speech a less earthly character than he has in daily life, he will be helped by beings from the angelic world. Rudolf Steiner said about eurythmy:

But if our everyday gesture is transformed into
articulated gesture or eurythmy, then that which
one sees when it is transformed into speech, what
flows from being to being, is actually that which the
archangels speak to each other.

In eurythmy the human being carries out gestures that correspond to speech in the world of the archangels:

So we actually accompany with an eminently
super-earthly element that which the poet wishes to
raise into the super-earthly, not by emphasising the
prosaic but by treating it in a pictorial, sculptural,
musical manner. It may appear a little eccentric
when we say eurythmy is the earthly image of the
speech of archangels.[24]

In his lectures Steiner also describes how in the present incarnation of the earth, luciferic beings are already leading us to ascend to the fifth and sixth principle in their microcosmic aspects, anticipating the macrocosmic developments that will take place properly on Jupiter and Venus. Christ, who is active on the earth, brings the great impulse of the macrocosmic 'I' so that the human or microcosmic 'I' can take it up and develop further.

And He (Christ) did not yet have the fifth
and six macrocosmic principles (the Spirit Self and
Life Spirit), for He will develop them so that He
can give them to humanity on Jupiter and Venus
... He entered into earthly evolution in such a way
that He did not possess a fifth, sixth and seventh
principle – just as humanity did not.[25]

It is important to study this lecture, to live intensively in what is said about the turning inward of the human soul to infinite depths, and there receiving the gifts of light and love from the Christ impulse.

In this context it is deeply significant that the meditation from the third scene of *The Portal of Initiation*, 'Light's weaving essence...', was chosen by Rudolf and Marie Steiner as the opening piece for the performance in Zürich on February 24, 1919, the first public performance of eurythmy outside of Dornach. Steiner called the meditation 'Words to the Spirit and to Love'. From the outset, eurythmy was presented in its deepest being as the new mystery art for our time for an audience who were mainly non-anthroposophists (see p. 96).

These words of Rudolf Steiner, along with the transformed verse found at the end of the seventh scene, if repeatedly studied and worked with, will most certainly help us progress in our struggle for understanding and deeper spiritual experience.

Only in the very distant future will Spirit Self and Life Spirit reach their true, complete and independent human development. On Jupiter, Christ will develop the fifth macrocosmic principle and on Venus the sixth macrocosmic principle so that he can give them to human beings. According to Steiner he will also:

> ...make people more inward ... more humble.
> The luciferic spirits will lead human beings beyond themselves and make them clever ... but will also give them a certain haughtiness, will teach them that they can become superhuman already during Earth evolution.[26]

Rudolf Steiner drew our attention to this danger as eurythmists of becoming arrogant when he said:

> Eurythmy is indeed something that must make its appearance in human evolution at this time; but there is no call for pride, for at present it can be a

mere babbling compared with what it will become in the future.[27]

The study of the numerous lectures Steiner gave on the development of human beings toward their higher nature is of great importance to eurythmists, both those who are studying the art and those who are already teaching or performing it on stage. The high aim that Steiner placed before us, to faithfully present through movement an image of the heavenly archetype of the human being, obliges us to undertake such many-sided, tireless study.

With poets of various nationalities we find quite a lot that hints at the experience of the higher nature of the human being described more or less faithfully. Take, for example, Goethe's poem 'The Wanderer's Storm Song', which begins 'Whom you do not leave, Genius...'. At one time we had given ourselves a great deal of trouble to make a eurythmy composition for this. We created complicated forms for the countless figures from the divine world that appear in the poem and tried them out on the stage in the Carpenter's Shop. It was very difficult for us. Rudolf Steiner looked at what we had done, then drew a form for only three figures. These forms appeared to me as a revelation of the relationship of the I to the two higher members of the human being.

Introductory form

I   A, C, H, A, C, H
II   D, O, S, D, O, S
II   M, I, L, M, I, L

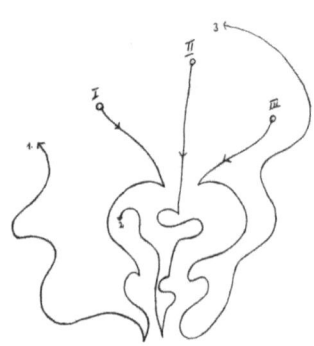

Until the fourth verse

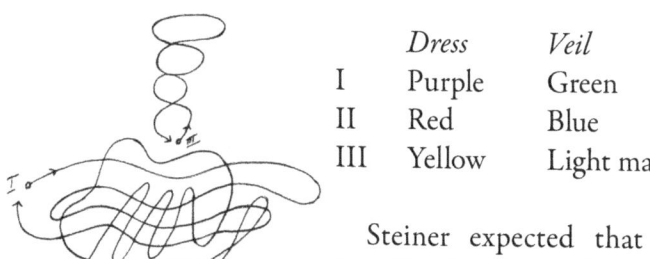

	Dress	Veil
I	Purple	Green
II	Red	Blue
III	Yellow	Light mauve

Steiner expected that what he offered in his work would be studied in order for it to become inner experience. He expressly recommended this in one of his lectures in which he built up a chart showing the development of the I and the other members of the human being, their connection to beings of the higher hierarchies, and their evolution from the distant past to the far distant future, from Old Saturn to Vulcan.[28] This diagram combined and made visible the contents of his various lecture cycles, and he encouraged his listeners to do the same.

> You just have to make the effort to do more than simply read the lectures one after another in sequence; but really try to make connections between the things that have been said ... And it is very useful to do this, because by working through the material offered in the lecture cycles, you move from an external reception of the material to an inner reworking of it. This inner reworking has genuine value for any true forward progress.[29]

To make similar schemes or tables for eurythmy requires intensive study of the fundamentals, as well as unceasing devotion toward developing a eurythmy technique.

Another question can arise in wrestling with this problem. Is it possible, already in our present incarnation, to have experiences of that world in which the union of the two higher principles of the human being take place? Steiner explained that present day humanity cannot consciously experience this future world, in which they now only pass through during sleep:

> And the world we then enter between falling asleep and waking up is a world of the future; therefore, we cannot perceive it. It is the world into which our earth will be transformed in those stages of development I have called Jupiter, Venus, and Vulcan, in my book *An Outline of Occult Science*. Thus, we modern people who are drilled to think intellectually live in nothingness when we are sleeping. We *are* not nothing, as I have to stress again and again, but we *live in nothingness* because we cannot yet experience the world we live in, which is the world of the future; it is as yet a nothing to us.[30]

Will it be different if one takes up anthroposophical thoughts? Not if one only receives them passively into one's thoughts. However, if one comes to experience anthroposophical truths not only passively, not only intellectually, but in a way that transforms one's whole being, then one can pour the realities experienced in sleep with strength of will into the thoughts of life when awake:

> People who want to be anthroposophists – and not simply accept anthroposophical thoughts passively but really assimilate them – must pour what they have been during their dreamless sleep into the pure thoughts of anthroposophy with the help of their strong will. Those people will then have reached the first stage of what we can legitimately call clairvoyance. Then they live clairvoyantly in the thoughts of anthroposophy.[31]

This need to assimilate anthroposophical truths for ourselves, to work on them with inner intensity and make them our own, calls to mind the words of Goethe that I quoted at the beginning of this chapter:

> The things that we inherit come alone
> To true possession by the spirit's toil.[32]

It is this earnest spirit's toil, by which we can make our own the wisdom Rudolf Steiner brought to us from the spiritual world, and which I pursued through my work with eurythmy, that I wish to encourage in the reader with my words.

Endnotes

1912–13: Foundations and Beginnings

1. On physical culture in education among the Greeks and modern peoples, see *Human Values in Education* (CW310), Rudolf Steiner Press, UK 2005, lecture of July 24, 1924.
2. From the essay 'Das Goetheanum in seinen zehn Jahren (Ten Years of the Goetheanum)', in *Der Goetheanumgedanke inmitten der Kulturkrisis der Gegenwart: Gesammelte Aufsätze aus der Wochenschift 'Das Goetheanum' 1921–1925 [The Goetheanum-Idea in the Middle of the Cultural Crisis of the Present: Collected Essays from the Periodical 'Das Goetheanum', 1921–1925] (GA36)*.
3. *Four Mystery Dramas* (CW14), SteinerBooks, USA 2007, p. 79f. Translated by Ruth and Hans Pusch.
4. Original drawings by Rudolf Steiner in *Eurythmy, Its Birth and Development* (CW277a), Rudolf Steiner Press, UK 2015, p. 22. This dance was nevertheless performed as I have drawn it.
5. See *Four Mystery Dramas*.
6. *Secrets of the Threshold* (CW147), Anthroposophic Press, USA 1987.
7. *Eurythmy: Its Birth and Development* (CW277a), Anastasi Ltd, UK 2015, p. 52.
8. Ibid.
9. Ibid. See also lecture of October 28, 1909, 'The Nature and Origin of the Arts'.
10. Ibid, p. 53
11. *Inner Reading and Inner Hearing* (CW156), Steiner Books, USA 2008, p. 81.
12. *Eurythmy: Its Birth and Development* (CW277a), p. 55.

1913–15: Building Up

1. See lecture of October 11, 1913, 'The Transformation of Earthly Forces into Clairvoyant Faculties'.
2. Rudolf Steiner's statement that white eurythmy robes should be worn by adults and light green ones by children was carefully observed in the first years of our work in Dornach.
3. *Man in the Light of Occultism, Theosophy and Philosophy* (CW137), Rudolf Steiner Press, UK 1964. See lecture of June 12, 1912.

4. *Human and Cosmic Thought* (CW151), Rudolf Steiner Press, UK 2015.
5. According to Steiner the twelve worldviews are Materialism, Sensationalism, Phenomenalism, Realism, Dynamism, Monadism, Spiritism, Pneumatism, Psychism, Idealism, Rationalism and Mathematism. The seven soul moods are Gnosticism, Logicism, Voluntarism, Empiricism, Mysticism, Transcendentalism and Occultism.
6. *Human and Cosmic Thought*, p. 53.
7. Contained in *The Mystery of the Trinity* (CW214), SteinerBooks, USA 2016.
8. *Inner Reading and Inner Hearing* (CW156), lecture of October 7, 1914.
9. Ibid, p. 80f.
10. *Verses and Meditations*, Rudolf Steiner Press, UK 2004, p. 71.
11. See *Michael's Mission: Revealing the Essential Secrets of Human Nature* (CW194), Rudolf Steiner Press, UK 2015, lecture of December 14, 1919.
12. Contained in *Truth-Wrought Words* (CW40), SteinerBooks, USA 2010.
13. *The Festivals and their Meaning*, Rudolf Steiner Press, UK 2002, p. 267f. See also *Verses and Meditations*, p. 83.
14. *Anthroposophy in the Light of Goethe's* Faust (CW272), SteinerBooks, USA 2014, p. 148.
15. Ibid, p. 133.
16. Ibid, p. 148.
17. All quotes taken from: Goethe, Johann Wolfgang, *Faust: Part One* and *Faust: Part Two* (trans. Philip Wayne), Penguin, London (1949, 1959).
18. *Spirit as Sculptor of the Human Organism* (CW218), Rudolf Steiner Press, UK 2014, p. 213.
19. See *Four Mystery Dramas*, pp. 108–112. The scene was performed from the beginning until just before Johannes enters.
20. *Eurythmy: Its Birth and Development* (CW277a), p. 113.
21. *Rosicrucianism and Modern Initiation* (CW233a), Rudolf Steiner Press, UK 2020, p. 122.

1915–18: Expansion and Deepening

1. *Eurythmy: Its Birth and Development* (CW277a), p. 66f.
2. Translation by Marc Knight.
3. See *Eurythmy as Visible Singing* (CW278), Rudolf Steiner Press, UK 2019.
4. 'Das Goetheanum in seinen zehn Jahren (Ten Years of the Goetheanum)', in *Der Goetheanumgedanke inmitten der Kulturkrisis*

der Gegenwart: Gesammelte Aufsätze aus der Wochenschrift 'Das Goetheanum' 1921–1925* [*The Goetheanum-Idea in the Middle of the Cultural Crisis of the Present: Collected Essays from the Periodical 'Das Goetheanum', 1921–1925]* (GA36).
5. *Eurythmy: Its Birth and Development* (CW277a), p. 66f.
6. 'Das Goetheanum in seinen zehn Jahren (Ten Years of the Goetheanum)', in *Der Goetheanumgedanke inmitten der Kulturkrisis der Gegenwart: Gesammelte Aufsätze aus der Wochenschrift 'Das Goetheanum' 1921–1925* [*The Goetheanum-Idea in the Middle of the Cultural Crisis of the Present: Collected Essays from the Periodical 'Das Goetheanum', 1921–1925]* (GA36).
7. Ibid.
8. Available as a single lecture in *The Alphabet: An Expression of the Mystery of Man*, Mercury Press, USA 1982.
9. See *Anthroposophy in the Light of Goethe's Faust* (CW272), SteinerBooks, USA 2014, and *Goethe's Faust in the Light of Anthroposophy* (CW273), SteinerBooks, USA 2016.

1918–19: Stepping Out in Public

1. *Eurythmy as Visible Speech* (CW279), Rudolf Steiner Press, UK 2019.
2. See *Colour* (CW291), Rudolf Steiner Press, UK 2005, pp. 80–89.
3. *The Bhagavad Gita and the West* (CW142/146), SteinerBooks, USA 2009.
4. *The Mystery of the Trinity* (CW214), p. 151.
5. Contained in *Eurythmie: Die Offenbarung der sprechenden Seele* [*Eurythmy: Revelation of the Speaking Soul*] (GA277).
6. Matt 18:3.
7. It has not been possible to find a precise attribution for this quote, but see *Ancient Myths and the New Isis Mystery*, Anthroposophic Press, USA 1994, especially the lecture of January 6, 1918.
8. See *Four Mystery Dramas* (CW14).
9. *The Karma of Vocation* (CW172), SteinerBooks, USA 2020. See lecture of November 6, 1916.
10. Seven of the sixteen lectures given in this series, including the fourth one referred to here, can be found in *Ancient Myths and the New Isis Mystery*. See lecture of January 8, 1918.
11. *Toward Imagination* (CW169), SteinerBooks, USA 1998, p. 49f.
12. *The Spiritual Hierarchies and the Physical World* (CW110), SteinerBooks, USA 2008, p. 101. Other lecture cycles that touch on the subject of the twelve senses include *Man in the Light of Occultism, Theosophy and Philosophy* (CW137) and *Human and Cosmic Thought* (CW151).
13. *Twelve Moods*, Mercury Press, USA 2012, p. 8ff.
14. *Toward Imagination* (CW169), p. 117.

15. *Twelve Moods*, p. 9f.
16. Ibid, p. 7f.
17. *Faust – Part Two*, p. 25.

1919–24: In the House of the Word

1. *Speech and Drama* (CW282), SteinerBooks, USA 2007. Marie Steiner's introduction, which is considerably longer in the German language, was shortened for the English edition, leaving out much that Kisseleff quotes here and elsewhere.
2. *Soul Economy and Waldorf Education* (CW303), Steiner Books, USA 2014, lectures of December 28 and 30, 1921.
3. *Art as Seen in the Light of Mystery Wisdom* (CW275), Rudolf Steiner Press, UK 2010. Lecture of December 29, 1914.
4. *Speech and Drama* (CW282). See note 1 to this chapter for an explanation of the introduction.
5. *Man and the World of the Stars* (CW219), SteinerBooks, USA 1982. Lecture of December 31, 1922.
6. See *World History and the Mysteries in the Light of Anthroposophy* (CW233), Rudolf Steiner Press, UK 1997, lecture of December 31, 1923; and *Rosicrucianism and Modern Initiation: Mystery Centres of the Middle Ages* (CW233a), Rudolf Steiner Press, UK 2020. Lecture of April 22, 1924.
7. *Art as Seen in the Light of Mystery Wisdom* (CW275), Rudolf Steiner Press, UK 2010, p. 121.
8. Contained in *Bühnenkunst am Goetheanum*, No. 4, Easter 1937.
9. *Eurythmy as Visible Singing* (CW278), Rudolf Steiner Press, UK 2019, and *Eurythmy as Visible Speech* (CW279), Rudolf Steiner Press, UK 2019.

1924–27: Rudolf Steiner's Death – A Turning Point in My Life

1. *The Gospel of St John and Its Relation to the Other Gospels* (CW112), Anthroposophic Press, USA 1948, p. 155f.
2. *The Arts and Their Mission* (CW276), SteinerBooks, USA 1998, p. 97.
3. *Speech and Drama* (CW282), p, 253.
4. Ibid, p. 7.

1927–39: Paris – Studio rue Huyghens and the École Rudolf Steiner

1. *Foundations of Esotericism* (CW93a), Rudolf Steiner Press, UK 2019. Lecture of October 31, 1905.
2. *Eurythmy as Visible Speech* (CW279), p. 86.

3. *Vergangenheits- und Zukunftsimpulse im sozialen Geschehen. Die geistigen Hintergründe deer sozialen Frage, Band II* [*Impulses of the Past and Future in Social Occurrences. The Spiritual Background of the Social Question, Volume 2*] (GA190). The lecture of March 29, 1919 can be found in the pamphlet *The Time-Sequence and Spiritual Foundation of Threefolding*, Mercury Press, USA 1998.
4. *The Genius of Language* (CW299), Anthroposophic Press, USA 1995, p. 46.
5. *Speech and Drama* (CW282), p. 43f.
6. See *Eurythmy as Visible Speech* (CW279), p. 159.
7. *Eurythmy as Visible Singing* (CW278), p. 40f.
8. *Eurythmy as Visible Speech* (CW279), p. 64.
9. Ibid, p. 64.
10. Ibid, p. 53.
11. *Eurythmy as Visible Singing* (CW278), p. 39.
12. *Aus schicksalstragender Zeit* [*From Destiny-Burdened Times*] (GA64), lecture of October 29, 1914.
13. *Foundations of Esotericism* (CW93a), lecture of September 26, 1905.
14. *The Spiritual Guidance of the Individual and Humanity* (CW15), SteinerBooks, USA 1991, p. 37.
15. *Ancient Myths and the New Isis Mystery* (CW180), lecture of January 8, 1918.
16. *Eurythmy as Visible Speech* (CW279), p. 86.
17. Ibid, p. 85f.
18. *Speech and Drama* (CW282), p. 371f.
19. *Eurythmy as Visible Speech* (CW279), p. 43.
20. *Ancient Myths and the New Isis Mystery* (CW180), lecture of January 5, 1918.
21. Ibid, lecture of January 8, 1918.

The Future of Eurythmy

1. *Faust: Part One*, p. 53.
2. *Building Stones for an Understanding of the Mystery of Golgotha* (CW175), Rudolf Steiner Press, UK 2015, p. 22.
3. See *Death as Metamorphosis of Life* (CW182), SteinerBooks, USA 2008, p. 149f. See also *Life Between Death and Rebirth* (CW140), Anthroposophic Press, USA 1968, p. 100f.
4. *Eurythmy as Visible Speech* (CW279), p. 53.
5. *Art as Seen in the Light of Mystery Wisdom* (CW275), p. 41.
6. *Michael's Mission* (CW194), Rudolf Steiner Press, UK 2015, p. 205.
7. *Man in the Light of Occultism, Theosophy and Philosophy* (CW137), p. 90.
8. Ibid, p. 91f.

9. *Kunst und Lebensfragen im Lichte der Geisteswissenschaft* [*The Questions of Art and Life in the Light of Spiritual Science*] (GA162), lecture of July 17, 1915.
10. *Man in the Light of Occultism, Theosophy and Philosophy* (CW137), p. 108f.
11. *The Gospel of Luke* (CW114), Anthroposophic Press, USA 1964, p. 200.
12. *Eurythmy As Visible Speech* (CW279), p. 45.
13. Ibid, p. 57.
14. Ibid.
15. Ibid, p. 52.
16. *Artistic Sensitivity as a Spiritual Approach to Knowing Life and the World* (CW161), SteinerBooks, USA 2018, p. 6.
17. *Art as Seen in the Light of Mystery Wisdom* (CW275), p. 41.
18. Ibid, p. 50.
19. *Building Stones for an Understanding of the Mystery of Golgotha* (CW175), p. 188f.
20. *The Gospel of John* (CW103), Anthroposophic Press, USA 1962, p. 179.
21. *Building Stones for an Understanding of the Mystery of Golgotha* (CW175), p. 217f.
22. Ibid, p. 218.
23. *Esoteric Christianity and the Mission of Christian Rosenkreutz* (CW130), Rudolf Steiner Press, UK 2000, p. 191f.
24. From speeches given on July 8 and 9, 1923, contained in *Eurythmie: Die Offenbarung der sprechenden Seele* [*Eurythmy: Revelation of the Speaking Soul*] (GA277).
25. *Esoteric Christianity and the Mission of Christian Rosenkreutz* (CW130), p. 200.
26. Ibid, p. 201.
27. *Art as Seen in the Light of Mystery Wisdom* (CW275), p. 41.
28. *Artistic Sensitivity* (CW161), p. 3.
29. Ibid, p. 10.
30. *Earthly Knowledge and Heavenly Wisdom* (CW221), Anthroposophic Press, USA 1981, p. 26.
31. Ibid, p. 30.
32. *Faust: Part One*, p. 53.

Selected Bibliography

Steiner, Rudolf, *Architecture as Peacework: The First Goetheanum, Dornach, 1914* (CW287), SteinerBooks, USA 2017.
—, *Architecture, Sculpture, and Painting of the First Goetheanum* (CW288), SteinerBooks, USA 2017.
—, *The Arts and Their Mission* (CW276), SteinerBooks, USA 1998.
—, *Art as Seen in the Light of Mystery Wisdom* (CW275), Rudolf Steiner Press, UK 2010.
—, *Artistic Sensitivity as a Spiritual Approach to Knowing Life and the World* (CW161), SteinerBooks, USA 2018.
—, *The Early History of Eurythmy* (CW277c), SteinerBooks, USA 2015.
—, *Eurythmy as Visible Singing* (CW278), Rudolf Steiner Press, UK 2019.
—, *Eurythmy as Visible Speech* (CW279), Rudolf Steiner Press, UK 2019.
—, *Eurythmy: Its Birth and Development* (CW277a), Anastasi Ltd, UK 2015.
—, *Four Mystery Dramas* (CW14), SteinerBooks, USA 2007.
—, *The Genius of Language* (CW299), Anthroposophic Press, USA 1995.
—, *Speech and Drama* (CW282), SteinerBooks, USA 2007.
—, *Truth-Wrought-Words* (CW40), SteinerBooks, USA 2010.
—, *Twelve Moods*, Mercury Press, USA 2012.
—, *Verses and Meditations*, Rudolf Steiner Press, UK 2004.

Index

Abels, Joan 59
ahrimanic beings (in dance) 17–19
Apollonian Eurythmy 77

Baumann-Dolfuss, Elisabeth 121
'Behold the sun' (verse) 44–46
Belyi, Andrei 149

Carpenter's Shop 40f
Carson, Louise 31
children's eurythmy 104f, 108–10, 153f
Chinese language 171
Clason, Louise 65, 114, 124
colours in eurythmy 106
consonants in evolution sequence 36–38, 172–74
consonants and zodiac 115–17
Coroze, Paul 151–53

dance, sylph and gnome 21f
dance of the stars 39f
dance of luciferic and ahrimanic thought-beings 17–19
decan (10° division of zodiac) 177–80
Deventer-Wolfram, Erna von 25, 76f
Dietschi, Frau 31
disruptions at performances 122f, 124
Dolfuss, Elisabeth *see* Baumann-Dolfuss, Elisabeth
dress, eurythmy 94
Dubach-Donath, Annemarie 35, 77
Duncan, Isadora 141, 156

Egyptian language, ancient 171
Elisabeth Dollfuss-Baumann 76f
Ellram, Bertha 93, 114
English, sounds and eurythmy in 159, 166
eurythmy, first lecture about 41f
— course, first (Basel, Sep 1912) 20f
— —, second (Aug–Sep 1915) 84
— figures 131f
— training, beginnings 139f

Faust, scenes from 49–61, 90–94
French, sounds and eurythmy in 157–61, 163f, 166f
Froböse, Edwin 58

Goetheanum, as House of the Word 134–38
—, burning of 86, 132f
— stage 128–31
Grimm, Hermann 41

Hansi, Villa (early beginnings) 32f
Harris, Lilla 31
Hollenbach, Hendrika 80
houses (of zodiac) 178–80
humoresques 87f

India, ancient 172

Japanese language 171
John, Prologue of Gospel of 63f
Joseph (in Christmas play) 61
Jura, Hotel (early beginnings) 32

Kimball-von Baravalle, Ilse 95
Kisseleff, Tatiana 2, 9, 11, 76, 95
Klug-Schilbach, Erika 144
Kühne, Walter 31

Leinhaus-von Sonclar, Flossie 95
lemurs (in Faust) 61
lighting for eurythmy 128
Lord's Prayer 62–64
luciferic beings (in dance) 17–19

Maier-Smits, Lory 20, 25, 76f
Mauthner, Fritz 25
May, Walo von 97
microcosmic dance 88f
Mikhailovich, Grand Duke Alexander 151
Milscher, Käthe 65, 114
moods, twelve 117–19
Morgenstern, Christian 41, 79
Mystery Dramas and eurythmy 180–82
Mystery Drama seals 75

Nietzsche, Friedrich 26

Pals, Leopold van der 86, 93, 97, 124
Papoff, Wladimir 31
Pater Noster 62–64
Pfauen Theatre, Zürich 96–103
planets and vowels 114f
Portal of Initiation 64–74
Preludes 80, 87
public performances 96–103
Pyle, William Scott 138
Pyle-Waller, Mieta 31, 35, 39, 57, 77, 79, 106, 125, 138

Ricardo, Gracia 31
Rihouët-Coroze, Simone 151, 154, 156
Russian, sounds and eurythmy in 159–70

Sauerwein, Alice 156
Scholl, Mathide 31
Schultz, Joachim 177
Schuurman, Max 79, 86
Siedlecka, Wiga 31
Siver, Marie von *see* Steiner, Marie
Siver, Olga von 31
Smits, Lory *see* Maier-Smits, Lory
Solovyov, Vladimir 141
Speech and Drama course (Sep 1924) 136
Steffen, Albert 143
Steiner, Marie *passim,* 35
—, on tour 122–27
Steiner, Rudolf *passim,* 35
—, as actor 60f
Stuten, Jan 57, 86, 124
sylph and gnome dance 21f

Thesbians (actors' group) 146
tone eurythmy 77–82
touring performances 122–27
twelve moods 117–19

Unger-Palmer, Ruth 65

vowels, early forms for 26–30
—, expressing 43
— and planets 114f

Waller, Mieta *see* Pyle-Waller, Mieta
'Where outer senses' (verse) 46–49
White Room in Goetheanum 83–86
Whitsun verse 46–49
witches and warlocks cosumes 90f
World Clock 174–78

Zinovsky, Adina 32f
zodiac, gestures for 82
— and consonants 115–17

You may also be interested in...

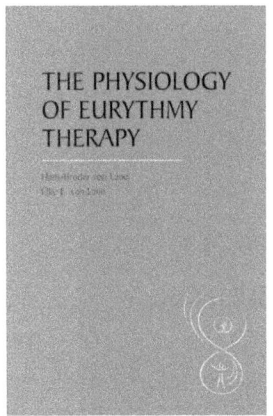
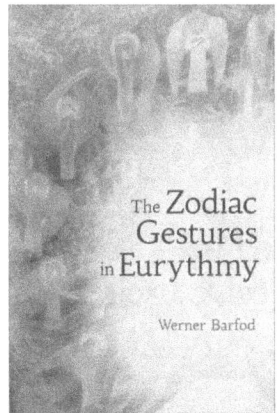
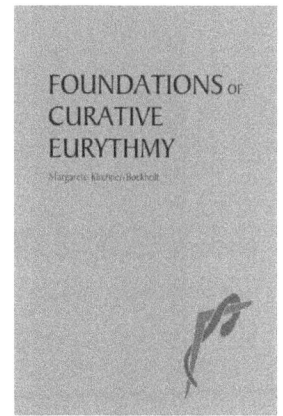
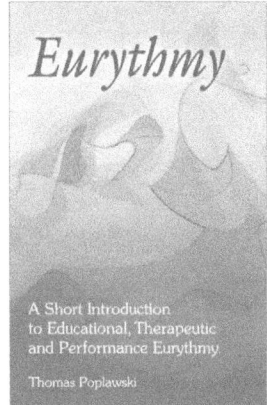
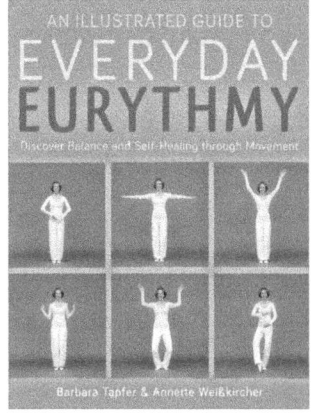

florisbooks.co.uk

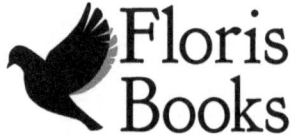

For news on all our **latest books**,
and to receive **exclusive discounts**,
join our mailing list at:

florisbooks.co.uk

Plus subscribers get a FREE book
with every online order!

We will never pass your details to anyone else.